8/11

KNACK
MAKE IT EASY

ABS

ABS

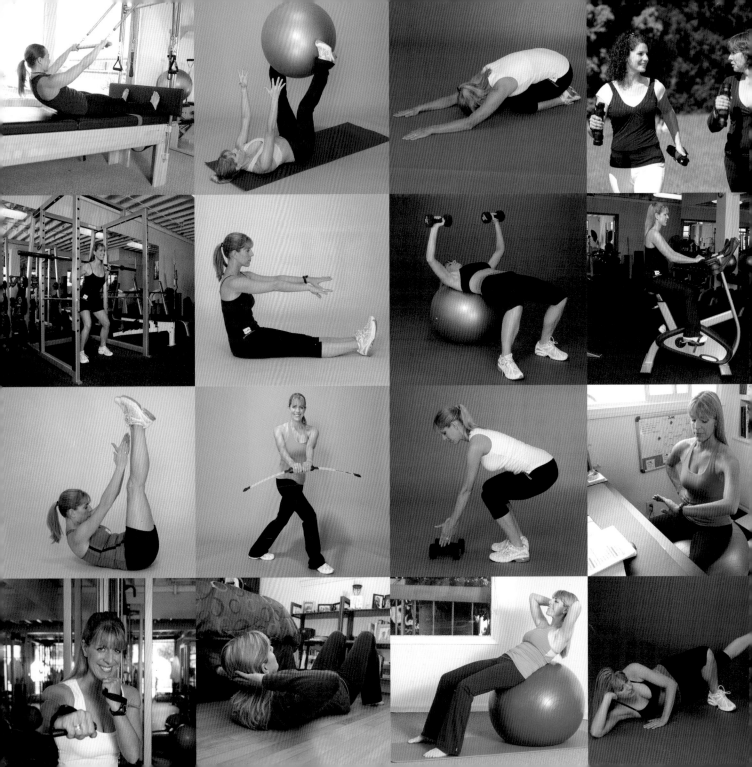

KNACK

ABSOLUTE ABS

Routines for a Fit & Firm Core

JJ Flizanes

Photographs by Starla Fortunato

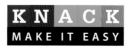

Guilford, Connecticut
An imprint of Globe Pequot Press

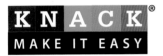

Copyright © 2011 by Morris Book Publishing, LLC

Editorial Director: Cynthia Hughes
Editor: Lara Asher
Project Editor: Tracee Williams
Cover Design: Paul Beatrice, Bret Kerr
Interior Design: Paul Beatrice
Layout: Melissa Evarts
Cover Photos by Starla Fortunato
Interior Photos by Starla Fortunato with the exception of those on page 2: © Patrick Hermans | Shutterstock; page 3: © Patrick Hermans | Shutterstock; page 4 (right): © SvetikD | Shutterstock; page 11 (left): © Springoz | Shutterstock; page 16 (left): © Monika Wisniewska | Shutterstock; page 16 (right): © Sebastian Kaulitzki | Shutterstock; page 17 (left): © iDesign | Shutterstock; page 23 (left): © baldari | Shutterstock; page 48: Illustration by Ian Adamson © Globe Pequot Press; page 54 (left): © Patrick Hermans | Shutterstock; page 93 (left): © Oguz Aral | Shutterstock; page 116 (right): © Patrick Hermans | Shutterstock; page 159 (left): © Sebastian Kaulitzki | Shutterstock; page 207 (left): © Michael Siegmund | Shutterstock; page 208 (left): © Yellowj | Shutterstock; page 211 (left): © Christy Thompson | Shutterstock; page 211 (right): © Victor Shova | Shutterstock; page 217 (right): © charlotteLake | Shutterstock.

The following manufacturers/names appearing in *Knack Absolute Abs* are trademarks:
ASICS®; Bodyblade®; Daiya™; FreeMotion™; Gymnastik®; Harbinger®; lucy®; The Paleo Diet™; Precor EFX 544®; RESTORE® CLOTHING; Skype™; Spinning®; StairMaster®; Star Trac®; Styrofoam™

Library of Congress Cataloging-in-Publication Data

Flizanes, J.J.
  Knack absolute abs : routines for a fit & firm core / J.J. Flizanes ; photographs by Starla Fortunato.
    p. cm.
  ISBN 978-1-59921-947-9
  1. Abdomen--Muscles. 2. Abdominal exercises. 3. Physical fitness. I. Fortunato, Starla. II. Title.
  GV508.F54 2011
  613.7'1886--dc22

                                                    2010041107

Printed in China

10 9 8 7 6 5 4 3 2 1

This book is dedicated to my husband Brian Albers, our future and our family. I wrote this with you in mind and in my heart.

Acknowledgments

I had no idea how much work could go into writing a book like this and I am grateful to many people for making it happen. First off, thank you to my sponsors Bodyblade, lucy, and RESTORE CLOTHING—you helped me look good! Thank you to Maria Ravis of El Segundo Acupuncture, Jeanne Peters and Dr. Allen Peters of Nourishing Wellness, Tracy Coe of Body & Mind Coe-Dynamics Pilates Studio, Russ Samuels of RJS Fitness, Adoley Odunton of Healthier Living, Josh Schyler and the crew at Every Angle Media, and Starla Fortunato and all of her assistants from Starla Fortunato Photography. A big thanks goes out to Jennifer Kwon, my friend and makeup artist who provided much more than makeup on this project—I appreciated your support. I want to acknowledge the National Academy of Sports Medicine and the Resistance Training Specialist Program for providing me with the foundation of knowledge that I use every day when creating fitness training programs. A big thank you to everyone at Globe Pequot; Lara Asher, Tracee Williams, and Katie Benoit. I could not have done it without you. All of this would not have been possible without my wonderful literary agent Julie Hill—I am so grateful to be working with you. Thank you to my clients and friends for the support I got during this long and often stressful process. Special thanks to Macarena Bianchi, Kelly Abrajano, Bibi Goldstein, Cathy Alessandra, Jeanne Peters, Jenny Buckles, Midge Ebben, and Valerie Flizanes for emotional support during this journey. Thank you to my family for permission to appear in the book; Brian Albers, Gus Flizanes, Valerie Flizanes, Brian Flizanes, and Helen Ciavarra. I am proud to have you as my family and want the world to know! I am a very lucky woman to have such amazing parents who have supported me in everything I do since the day I was born. I owe you everything and then some. You are truly special people and amazing parents. I love you very much and thank you from the bottom of my heart. In closing, I want to thank and acknowledge the support and love from my husband, Brian Albers. Without you, this book and my sanity could not have been possible. Thank you for everything you do to support my dreams, our future, our family and our life. I have been blessed to have manifested the perfect partner in a wonderful man who is a supportive and caring husband. I love you very much!

CONTENTS

INTRODUCTION

If you're like a lot of people, you're obsessed with your midsection, or core. This actually may be a good thing. After all, having excess weight around the middle waist is a risk factor for heart disease and diabetes. The extra weight also shifts your center of gravity, can put a strain on your lower back, and can leave your spine vulnerable to injury if your core muscles don't do their job. Clearly, you have some good reasons besides appearance to be concerned about your core.

Having a strong core also increases your strength in all your joints and muscles when you activate those muscles while doing daily activities or exercising any part of your body. But is it necessary to have a six-pack in order to achieve optimal health of your midsection and back? No. In fact if you have a six-pack but don't activate it during an exercise, you still put your back at risk of injury.

In this book you are going to focus on a fit and firm core that not only looks good but is also functional in its role in strength and stability in your body and life. My goals for you are to love your body, exercise, and feed it well, and celebrate every accomplishment you make no matter how big or small. We will focus on the abdominal region, but I want you to not lose focus on the bigger reason you bought this book. You want to be happy, love your body, and love your life. We can do that and begin today.

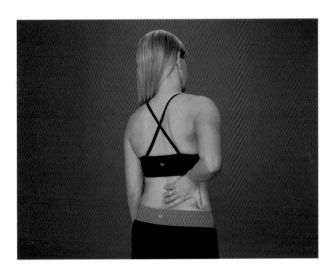

Conquering weight-loss resistance

This book may not offer the advice you're used to receiving. If you have watched infomercials for abs products, or have seen them advertised in newspapers or magazines, you know they often make unrealistic promises. They may say the product will do all the work for you or that you need only work 5 minutes a day to achieve great results. We as consumers are led to believe that the magic of a slim waist comes from outside of ourselves, as long as we use some complicated machine or take a pill.

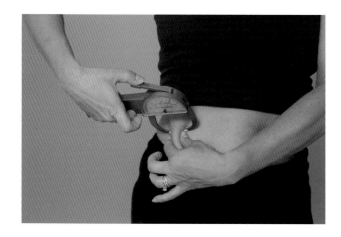

of them in this book. We will also address some mental and emotional factors that keep you stuck and prevent you from getting the results you desire.

This comprehensive book will address almost every area of your life, and we will work from both the inside out and the outside in. One factor that works wonders for one person may not be the same one that helps you. Be open to trying it all and doing so out of self-love and self-care.

Dietary changes

Treat your body like an experiment as you read through this book and implement the strategies. Take a food sensitivity test. See how your body responds to dietary changes. Since there are many factors that contribute to your success, I encourage you to journal your way through and have fun along the way. As with all health and fitness goals, there is really never an end point. Once you shed a few pounds, gain some strength and endurance, and feel better, you will want to maintain that and maybe even surpass it onto the next fitness level.

I wrote this book to help you understand that a fit and trim middle absolutely does not depend on just one thing. In fact, it depends on several different factors. For example, a huge part of trimming your waistline starts with the food you eat. So, if you have food sensitivities, you may find it very difficult to achieve your goals without addressing this problem. Another factor is water retention. Many people battle bloating and excess water retention that no cardio or resistance training alone can eliminate. These factors and others are part of something called weight-loss resistance. I am sure you know someone who does all the "right" things but cannot lose weight—it may even be you. There are several weight-loss resistance factors, and we will cover a few

I have had clients who love the changes in their health and body so much that they want to move on to more competitive goals like running a race, climbing a mountain, or doing a triathlon. But these athletic goals are not for

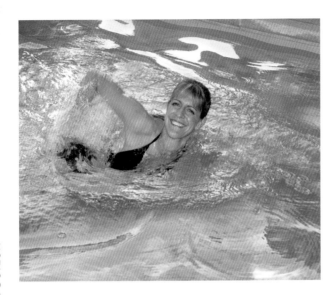

everyone, and there is no rush, so start where you are and take it one day at a time. I want you to use this book and the information in it to change your life forever, but it will take time and you will see results every step of the way if you commit to yourself and your journey.

Resistance training

In addition to learning about diet, you will also find out about the muscles of your core in great detail. After all, the more you understand how something works, the better you can work it. This is especially true for your body, and I want to educate you to your success. Remember that getting a fit and firm core is not as simple as doing a few core

exercises. If that were the case, we all would have achieved that already!

Another component of a fit and firm core is resistance training—for your abs as well as your whole body. Resistance training builds muscle, increases metabolism, and contributes to that tight, firm look that you want. But not all resistance training is created equal. You will learn proper form and technique, focusing on efficiency, safety, and effectiveness. If you feel you still need further instruction, I invite you to visit www.invisiblefitness.com for video instruction on some of the most popular exercises in this book.

Proper form and safety

Check with your doctor before starting an exercise program, and always choose safety first. The techniques I recommend for all exercises come from the point of view of protecting the body and getting results at the same time. Most people do not concern themselves with things like joint integrity until they get injured and it hurts to move.

Overextending yourself puts you at a risk of injury, and injuries set back your progress. Doing resistance training too fast with no body control also puts your joints and spine at risk for injury. So please always go slowly and think about what you are doing as you perform each exercise. Exercise can either speed up degeneration of your joints or slow it down, depending on your form and technique.

A foundation in science

I know you will be successful, and I look forward to hearing all about your journey. My twelve years in the fitness industry as both a trainer and educator have prepared me to share with you the latest information coupled with the foundation of science that governs it all. I know that sometimes fitness can look trendy and driven by fads, but as long as solid science is the foundation, exercise can be one of the greatest forms of medicine and healing.

Your body is complex and designed to move. With our technologically driven culture, it is more important than ever to make moving a priority every day. Computers take movement away from us, yet give us the freedom to be mobile. Whatever situation you are in, there is always freedom in creating even just 5- or 10-minute exercise routines to fit your life.

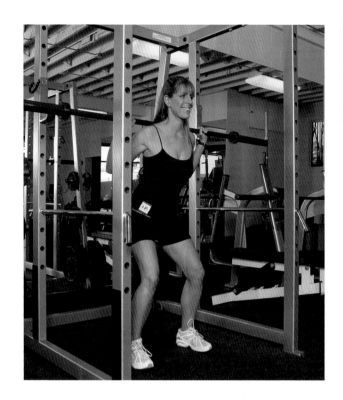

Invisible Fitness

I created Invisible Fitness to teach people that what they cannot see is often more important than what they can see. Your joints, heart, cardiovascular system, digestion, mind, emotions, and skeletal structure are affected daily by things that are invisible to you. Your heart rate increases when you walk fast or up a hill or stairs. Your muscles work harder to help you carry bags of groceries compared to when you have nothing in your hands. The invisible creates the visible.

When you begin this journey, remember to pay attention to all the invisible factors and benchmarks of your body and health, and be sure to monitor them throughout the program. When you know these things are changing, you can be sure that your body will follow.

You will be asked to expand your comfort zone in order to change, grow as a person, and expand into whom you really are. If it is time to shed a new skin, congratulations and enjoy the journey to the new you!

A FIRM & FIT CORE

Reducing body fat while increasing lean muscle will result in amazing abs

What is a fit and firm core? For each person the answer may vary, because we all have different goals! For some, it may mean having a visible six-pack and an athlete's remarkably low percentage of body fat. For others, it might just mean having a flat and firm midsection. Either way, the fact remains that in order to uncover your already sculpted abdominal

muscles, you must burn off some body fat through diet and exercise and add some lean muscle.

How you create your program will be based on your goals, and I do not want you to be intimidated by an idea or goal that is unrealistic or undesirable. Remember: Not everyone wants the same thing, so as you read through this book, pick

Your Abs

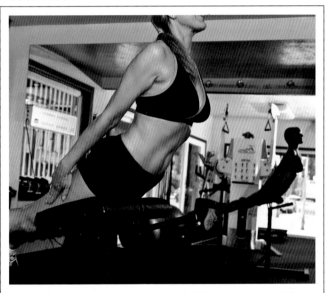

- Focusing on your abs can be a great place to start a program, because it gets you motivated to see results quickly.

- With a little effort and time, you can begin to feel the difference in strength and stability around your core with a few exercises a week.

- Building core strength is also important for posture, injury prevention, strength abilities for all joints, and supporting your back.

- Most ab exercises can be done anywhere!

Diet

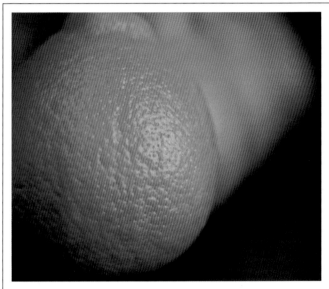

- What you eat is as important as how much you eat.

- Food is not only your fuel source for the body like gas in a car, but it also can enhance your metabolism and health or compromise them.

- With so many kinds of diets out there, we will focus on information about food and how your body responds to it.

- At least 50 percent of your results and health will be determined by the food you eat.

and choose what steps you want to incorporate first. You do not need to do everything all at once. I want to assure you that it is possible to get great results and it's not as hard as you may think.

Many people try to remove unwanted belly fat without success and then give up—feeling like exercise does not work. For those of you who have experienced this firsthand, we will cover some of the weight-loss resistance factors that could be hindering your progress. Some of these factors include hormones, food sensitivities, and sleep, and then of course there are effective diet and exercise, too. These factors make a big difference in your results, so I hope you will consider their impact and learn more about them.

Because you are reading this book, I know you are ready for some change in your body, and I can't wait to help you get there! Read the whole book, remember to pace yourself, surround yourself with support, and have fun in the process!

Exercise

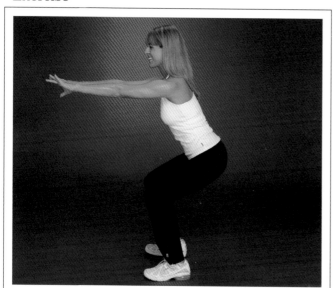

- Not all exercise is created equal. Just because you do something doesn't mean it's working.

- Building a personalized plan is imperative for your success. Every body is different.

- Use resistance training and cardio as your main tools to increase your metabolism and burn fat.

- Exercise is important for maintaining your health and will be crucial as you age if you want to stay vital.

Staying on Track

- Make sure to keep track of your program, progress, and accomplishments along the way to keep you motivated.

- Be accountable—it can make all the difference in sticking to your goals each week.

- Reward yourself with nonfood activities when you accomplish the next step.

- When life gets in the way, remember to get back on the surfboard to ride the wave again.

FOCUSING ON YOUR MIDDLE

Target muscles that make up your abs and build a program that fits your lifestyle

When most people start an exercise program, they do what they are told will work or focus on the latest "fad" without asking questions to determine if the program will fit their lifestyle and needs. They may go to the gym or sign up for an exercise class that meets two to three times a week for one hour. This may work for a while, but what happens when life gets busy? What happens when they must travel?

One of the most important things to consider when designing or choosing an exercise program is its longevity and flexibility. If your exercise routine does not fit into your lifestyle, you won't stick to it for long.

When I work with clients, I tell them that their goal should

Rectus Abdominis

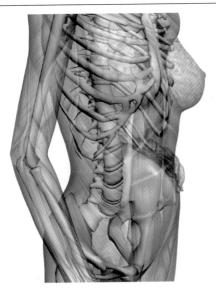

- Before you start to work your abs, you should know the different muscles that make up the area you want to work.

- The rectus abdominis is the muscle on the surface of the body in the front.

- This is usually the only muscle people really concentrate on because it is front and center on the body.

- Even though there are sections within the muscle, which have caused myths such as "upper and lower" abs, this is in fact one big muscle not two parts.

Internal and External Obliques

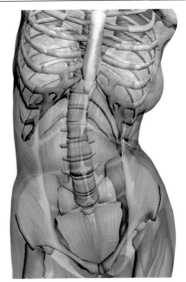

- People often call the fat that hangs over their jeans a spare tire or muffin top. This fat is actually covering the oblique muscles.

- Many people assume that twisting exercises will help tone this area, but some of these exercises are actually a waste of time and don't work.

- People can put their spine in danger by using too much force in a rotation exercise for the obliques, so it's really important to be careful.

be to build a program that both fits their body and schedule and can change and progress as they grow stronger. If you are a beginner exerciser, start slow and choose a few exercises to complete each week. If you are a regular exerciser now, compare your program to the suggestions in this book to fine-tune what you are doing. Sometimes one or two changes can make all the difference.

YELLOW LIGHT

If you are willing to change your lifestyle, try making small changes and see if you can maintain them for two to three months before making more. Most people change their lifestyle drastically for thirty to sixty days, and if they do not see the results they want, they fall back to their old habits and patterns. Health is a habit, not an event, so what you do consistently over time will make more difference than a short-term change in behavior.

Transversus Abdominis

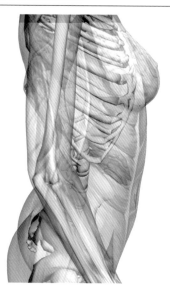

- This muscle is commonly referred to as the TVA.

- The deepest core muscle, you will not be able to see it on the surface of your body.

- Think of it as an internal belt around your spine and lower body.

- This muscle is activated automatically when you laugh or cough.

Quadratus Lumborum

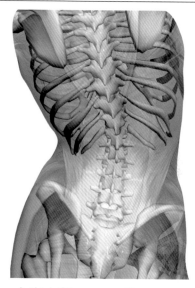

- Many people think if they "feel" something in their lower back that it means they have hurt themselves.

- The difference between pain and soreness is your clue to whether an injury or strain has occurred or if you have just worked your quadratus lumborum.

- There are many more muscles in the back that support the spine, but this one is most commonly misunderstood.

- Some people have a very tight lower back and can feel strain here when attempting to do abdominal work.

FACTS ABOUT SPOT REDUCING

Doing abs work alone will not ensure you obtain the midsection you want

One of the biggest myths out there when it comes to burning fat off your midsection is that you only need to work the abdominals. The muscles that make up the core are some of the most important because they support the spine, help with posture, and increase strength capabilities for the entire body. But only six groups of muscles make up the core! You have over three hundred muscles in your body that contribute to your overall metabolism.

In order to get fast and lasting results, you need to increase active tissue (muscle) in the whole body while reducing body fat and uncovering any weight-loss resistance along the way. Performing hundreds of crunches a day may help you feel

What Is Spot Reducing?

- Doing 100 sit-ups to shrink your middle is considered spot reducing when it's not followed by cardio, full-body training, or a proper diet.

- Twisting exercises to burn off love handles is another common yet ineffective attempt at spot reducing.

- You can exercise with goals in mind, but genetics do play a role in where the fat comes off and how you build muscle.

Liposuction

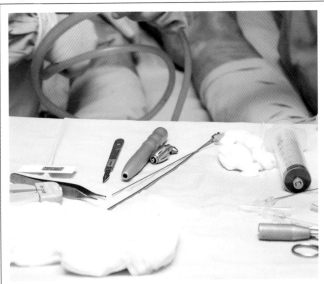

- The only way I know of to take off fat in specific areas is surgically through liposuction which is not guaranteed to work long-term.

- Some people who remove fat from one area gain more in a different area after surgery.

- While it is nice to think of removing a pocket of fat, you have to change your behavior and lifestyle to keep it off.

- Proper diet, exercise, and lifestyle change is the only way for long-term results with or without surgery.

like you are trimming down the fat around your middle, but without other components, you may not see results. When you use a free weight and do a bicep curl, do you expect the muscle to get smaller? No.

Most people expect it to become bigger, because of the added resistance. Doing abdominal work adds resistance to muscles in order to strengthen them, not shrink them. Your body chooses where the fat comes off once you engage in activities that require you to use your fat stores as energy. You can't decide for it. If that were true, we would all obtain fabulous results by focusing on one part at a time until it was the way we wanted it!

The best strategy for shaping your body combines efficient cardio to burn fat and resistance training to build muscle. And of course we can't forget about diet. You would not use a hammer alone to build an entire house, correct? You need many tools to help sculpt and shape your body from the inside out.

Creams

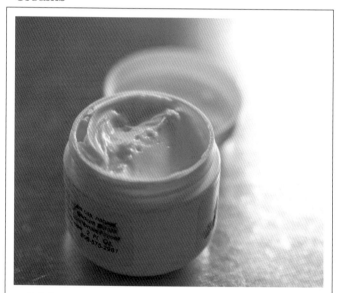

- Cellulite creams have become popular for reducing lines and wrinkles in your skin. But no cream will be able to "burn off fat" for you.

- If you invest in a cream, be sure to have realistic expectations about what it can do.

- You may improve the appearance of your skin, but fat removal is impossible.

- Try a change of diet with some exercise first to burn the fat which may make a greater difference in your skin.

Exercise

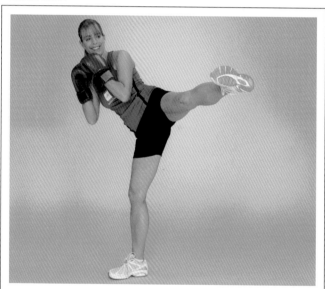

- Exercise can burn fat—this is true. But doing any exercise to target burning fat off of any one area is a myth.

- The best you can do is create a balanced program and target a section of muscle you want to build.

- Imagine doing a bicep curl to make your arms smaller. I hope you can see that this principle does not work.

- If exercising just the areas you want to reduce actually worked, wouldn't you have done it already?

TOTAL BODY PROGRAMMING
Exercise, stress management, and hormone regulation are all key to sculpting your abs

People often overlook stress as a factor in weight loss or weight gain. But stress can alter the body's chemistry, or hormones, creating an imbalance that can cause weight-loss resistance.

We have three major sets of hormones that regulate body chemistry. One set includes two adrenal hormones: cortisol

and DHEA. Cortisol is the "flight or fight" hormone. People especially needed this hormone in prehistoric times for survival. The hormone enables the body to flee or fight in the face of danger, and we still use this hormone today. However, because of our fast-paced, multitasked lives, many of us have elevated cortisol levels, and over time this creates what most

Meditation

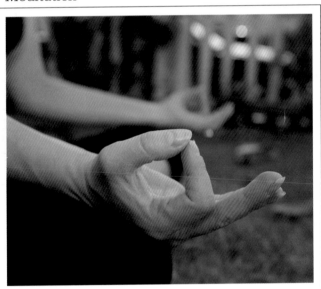

- Meditation is the practice of stillness and clearing your mind. You can do this by yourself or in a group.

- It can be as simple as 5 minutes a day where you focus on breathing. You can always increase the time to suit your preferences.

- Find a calm, serene environment and sit with your body upright in a comfortable position and eyes closed.

- Focus only on your breath as it goes in and out.

Yoga

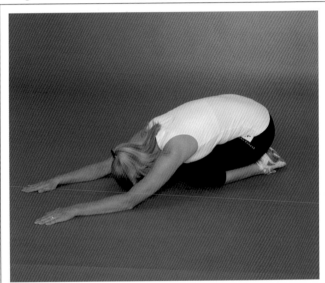

- There are many different kinds of yoga. Hatha yoga is great for beginners or those who want to receive the benefits of relaxation and stillness.

- For relaxation purposes, stay away from Bikram yoga, which uses heat to passively relax the body.

- This can be dangerous and does not serve the purpose of relaxation.

- Focus on your breathing, taking air slowly and fully into the body and releasing it gradually.

- Try incorporating a yoga class into your schedule.

people identify as "burn out," also known as adrenal fatigue.

Adrenal fatigue is the result of the combination of high cortisol levels and low DHEA levels. DHEA—often referred to as the "mother hormone"—supports all other hormones. If DHEA levels are low, it cannot help support the thyroid hormones or the sex hormones, the other two sets of hormones in the body, and over time this will cause weight-loss resistance.

ZOOM

Sleep and stress management are as important to your results as your diet and exercise, as they can regulate cortisol levels and not deplete your hormones. Adding rest and rejuvenation to your program is critical for long-term results. Meditation, yoga, hypnosis, and acupuncture are some ways to give your body the rest and stillness it needs to repair and replenish.

Hypnosis

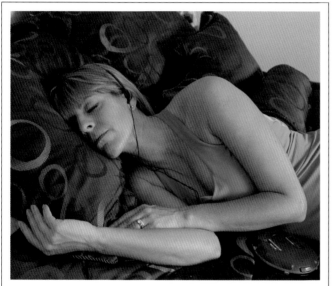

- Hypnosis is a powerful tool that can be as easy as putting on a headset before you go to sleep.

- Hypnosis targets the subconscious mind and reprograms it while you relax.

- You can find hypnosis for relaxation, weight loss, food cravings, and more.

- Hypnosis can have the same effects as guided meditation and bring you into deeper sleep, bring about slower and deeper breath, and slow your heart rate and blood pressure.

Acupuncture and Acupressure

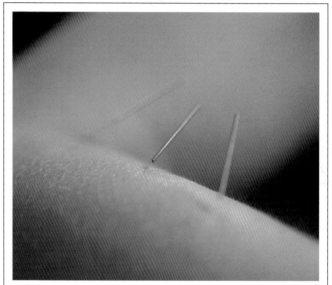

- Eastern medicine has been around for two thousand years, while Western medicine only two hundred.

- Acupuncture is the use of needles to activate energy meridians in the body to help with body ailments, digestion, and stress.

- Acupressure is the pressure point activated by touch without a needle.

- Incorporating acupuncture or acupressure into your health regimen can lower stress, monitor hormones, help with digestion, and a whole lot more!

TAKE THE QUIZ!

Find out where you are with your current diet and exercise program with this quiz

Where should you start? When beginning an exercise program, it is important to figure out where you are now, answer some basic questions, and create a personalized plan that will fit your lifestyle and goals. Too many times people kick off a new routine that is challenging to fit into their schedule, is uncomfortable on their body, or sets up unrealistic expectations that cause frustration and discouragement.

There are many aspects of building a program. The four main parts of a balanced plan are exercise, diet, rest, and support. When most people begin a diet or exercise program, they forget these other factors and wind up frustrated or overwhelmed. Aim to make this a lifestyle change and create

Choosing Exercises

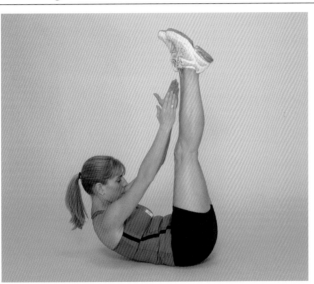

- What types of exercises are you incorporating into your program?

- What exercises have you tried in the past and what kind of results did you get?

- Will you do the exercises at home, in a gym, or outside? Will you exercise alone, with a friend, or in a class? Do you have all the proper tools to execute your exercises? What tools would you need on a weekly basis?

Dietary Changes

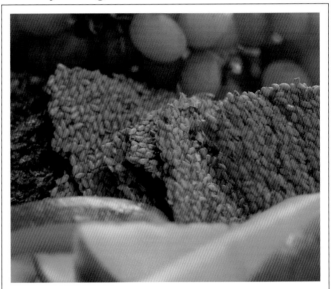

- What is the current state of your diet? What is the best and worst thing about it?

- List all of the changes you plan to make in your diet. Seeing them on paper will help you organize your thoughts and grocery list.

- What is the most important dietary change you can make that will make the biggest difference?

- Are you willing to make a lifestyle change or only a temporary change? Lifestyle changes have the most impact and tend to create lasting results.

a step-by-step plan. Answer the questions on these pages to help you assess where you are and what you need to do. Write down your answers in your journal. You may be excited to get started, and I want you to keep that excitement going by taking a few steps—but not too many steps. Too often, people do "all or nothing" but cannot sustain that for long. Let this be your first step in creating the body and health you want and doing it right!

YELLOW ● LIGHT

Be careful not to overanalyze numbers. Know where you are now, but don't allow yourself to get too caught up emotionally in the number on the scale. Take circumference measurements and a body composition test. Compare all the numbers every eight to twelve weeks for the most accurate information.

Rest and Rejuvenation

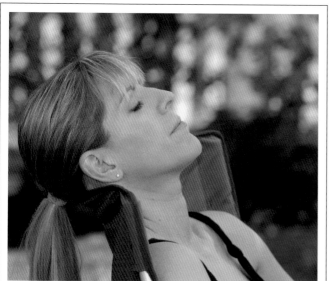

- Are you sleeping seven to nine hours each night? If not, what can you do to accomplish this?

- How many hours do you spend having fun or playing? This is important for mental and emotional balance and can help your results!

- Do you get acupuncture, massages, pedicures, or some other regular service that relieves stress?

- What is one thing you can do each day and week to recharge your body and mind?

Understanding Your Answers

- Identify what you want from your body and choose the appropriate exercises to get there.

- Diet makes up over 50 percent of your weight-loss and body-shaping results.

- The body repairs in rest mode, so make sure you get proper repair time.

- From your quiz, make a list of all the tools and support you will need for your program.

SET SOME GOALS!

Creating a plan must start with a clear and measurable vision

One of the main reasons why people get frustrated with their exercise or weight-loss program is because they have not set a clear measureable goal. I often speak at seminars, and I always ask people what it is they want to accomplish. The number one answer I get every time is to lose weight and be healthy. Now what does "be healthy" mean to you? How do you make a plan to be healthy? Would that plan be the same for everyone? Of course not. For some being healthy means lowering blood pressure and eating vegetables every day; for others it means being able to walk up the stairs easily.

The first step you must take on this journey is deciding where you want to be from where you are now. What does that look like? What does that feel like? Write it down. Once you have a clear picture, you can start to build a diet and exercise program to get you there. Think of it like a map. Without a map, you may get lost trying to go somewhere

Tape Measure

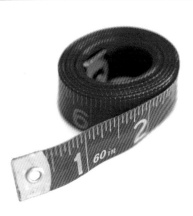

- Use a tape measure to measure different body parts so that you have a record of where you started. This will help show your progress.

- Many people lose inches before they lose weight. Knowing your measurements will let you know if you're on the right track.

- Measure your waist, legs, hips, arms, chest, neck, and calves. Keep a log and date it.

- Remeasure every six to eight weeks in the same location with the same equipment to ensure accuracy.

Body Fat

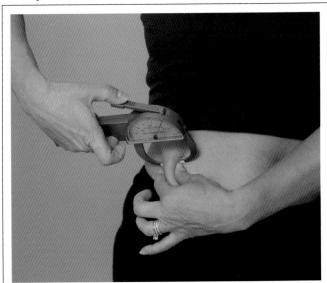

- There are many ways to test body fat. Hydrostatic weighing, skin calipers, bioimpedance, and tape measure are the most common. Hydrostatic weighing is done in a tank of water; bioimpedance uses an electric wave.

- Muscle burns calories; fat does not. Focus on lowering your body fat while increasing your lean muscle.

- To track progress, use the same equipment and method to test your body fat every eight to ten weeks.

- A fit and healthy range for women is 16 to 25 percent.

you have never been before. And after much trial and error, you may give up. Have a clear vision, set your goals, and create your map.

The Scale

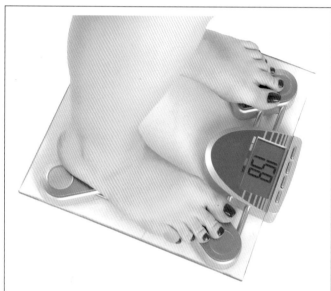

- The scale provides one number to consider. Know that your body weight can fluctuate every day.

- Weigh yourself once a month, not once a day. People abuse the scale by allowing themselves to be happy or sad by that number.

- To get a more complete reading of your progress, measure body fat too.

- Don't focus on your weight. If you loved the way you looked, would you really care what that number was?

Clothes

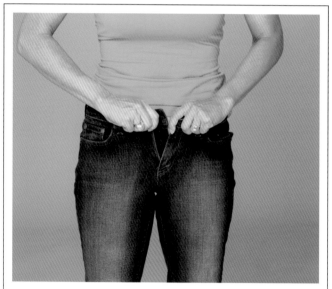

- Clothes can help you gauge your progress. Pick a few items to try on and set them aside for six to eight weeks. Try them on again before weighing or measuring.

- Choose clothes that are just a little too tight. Use this method for tracking your short-term results.

- It's more about how you feel than how you look. You might want to lose weight because you think it will make you happy. Choose to be happy now!

YOUR EXERCISE "STORY"

How to become someone who loves to exercise

Everyone has a "story" around food and exercise. You may be conscious of your story, or it may lie somewhere in your subconscious.

Did you know that 12 percent of your mind is conscious? These are the thoughts you are aware of. So of all the thoughts you have on a daily basis, you can hear only 12 percent of them. That means that 88 percent of your mind is subconscious, or is filled with thoughts that you are not aware of. Eighty-eight percent is a lot of thoughts that you cannot hear yourself think! We call the subconscious the basement of the mind. Yours was established between the time you were born until around age eight or nine. Just as in many homes, a lot of unwanted stuff gets stuffed in the basement.

Consciously you might say to yourself, "I know I should exercise." But subconsciously there is programming that simply

Start with the Conscious Mind

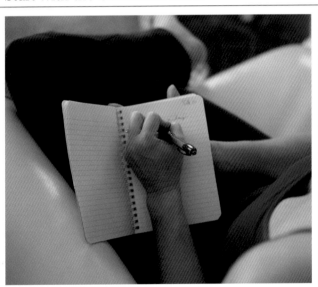

- Start by using your conscious mind and write down all the "excuses" you use to not exercise or to eat foods that are not the best choices.

- The things you write down are your "story." Identify where you can make small but impactful shifts in your internal discussions.

- Now write a new story. Spend 3 to 5 minutes with your eyes closed imagining life as you would like it to be and then write it down exactly that way.

Self-Hypnosis

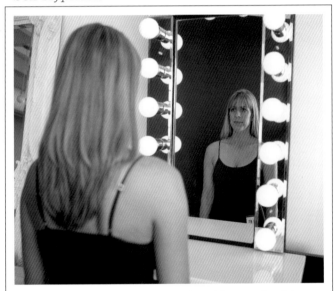

- Pick the most common excuse you use. Look in the mirror and say it aloud. Then for 5 minutes, name all the reasons why that is the most ridiculous thing you have ever heard.

- Say aloud, "That is the most ridiculous thing I have ever heard, because" and then fill in the blank. Doing this with a partner can accelerate the changes.

- Do this for three excuses you use on a weekly basis, and witness your mind and habits start to change!

does not want you to do it and has something else in mind. Even though you can get your mind to change the behavior for a period of time—we call this willpower—the subconscious mind acts like the undertow of the ocean and pulls you back into the water.

We all deal with this subconscious programming, but we are not necessarily aware of it. If you have been on many diets, or tried to be regular and consistent about exercise and failed, your subconscious mind is most likely to blame. Two of my favorite tools to use to help change this behavior are hypnosis and creative visualization. Hypnosis speaks to the subconscious mind and helps change your story, change your beliefs, and therefore change your habits. Talk therapy can be effective as well, but hypnosis is easier, faster, and sometimes much more pleasant! To get a free sample from my 6 Week Beach Body Program, visit www.6weekbeachbody.com.

While You Sleep

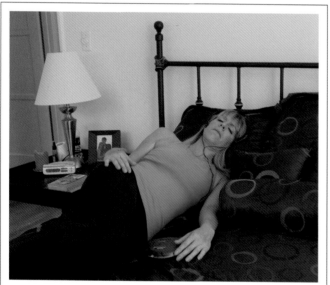

- One of the most effective ways to use hypnosis is to incorporate it as a daily ritual before bed.

- There are audiotapes for every subject, including "Getting Rid of Urges and Cravings," "Eat, Drink the Right Foods," "Exercising for Healthier Living," and more.

- Changing your habits at the deepest level makes changing your life and results easy.

- Remember that 88 percent of your mind is subconscious, so adding hypnosis can help you change your story more quickly!

Tips for Changing Your Story

- Identify your excuses so you can start reprogramming yourself.

- Notice your thoughts and practice choosing more supportive, positive thoughts to help you make diet and exercise a part of your everyday life.

- Use hypnosis on a regular basis to support these changes and accelerate your results.

- You are what you think you are!

13

THINKING THIN

Do you know how to "think thin?" Fit people think differently

Think thin! Your mindset is absolutely critical to your long-term success. How you think and what you focus on have everything to do with your ability to lose and maintain your weight loss. Have you ever heard that wealthy people think differently than poor people? It's the same with weight and health.

Thin people don't think, act, or have the habits of someone who is overweight. If you were to walk into their house and open the refrigerator and cupboards, they would look entirely different. Thin people can go out to a restaurant and enjoy having a salad even if everyone else is having pasta. They can take a bite of dessert and then put it down. They feel motivated to get up and exercise three or four times a week. They can go to a party and not binge on desserts and snack foods.

How do they do this? Well, there is a mindset that goes

Drink Plenty of Water

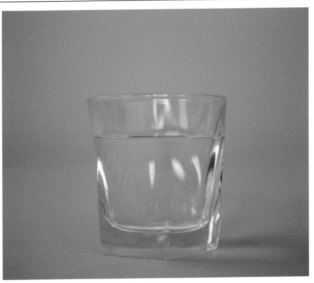

- Thinking thin involves simple but powerful changes, such as drinking water often. Thin people do not drink sodas or high-sugar drinks—they drink mostly water.

- Water makes up more than 55 percent of your body weight and is involved in every bodily function.

- Water is fresh, clean, and calorie free, and it replenishes the body and cells.

- Thin people crave water and imagine the refreshing feeling of drinking a cold glass of thirst-quenching goodness!

Get Moving!

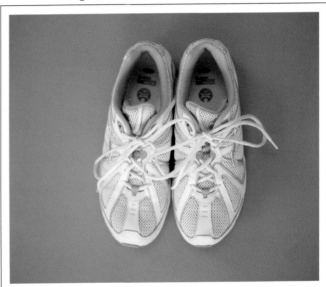

- Thin people own at least one good pair of athletic shoes or walking shoes. Thinking thin means acknowledging movement as exercise.

- Whether it's household chores, work, or a walk, they consider all movement to be exercise.

- Thin people are happy when they get in some exercise. They feel accomplished and a satisfaction from spending time taking care of their bodies.

- Thin people look forward to movement and even crave it. They do not like to be sedentary for long!

along with those behaviors. And when you have that mind-set, losing weight becomes easy and natural and you don't feel deprived. We use hypnosis and creative visualization to help change your mindset, and you can start today with 5 minutes of meditation. Clearing your mind allows you to make room for information from your subconscious.

I use the word thin to also describe fit and healthy. Some thin people are not necessarily fit or healthy. Being thin on the outside does not mean health on the inside. Anorexia and bulimia result in an unhealthy thin that is very dangerous and often deadly. As you read these pages, imagine "thinking thin" as the label for fit, healthy, balanced, and happy.

BRAIN POWER

Eat More Salad

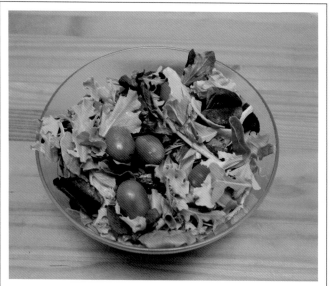

- Thin people love eating sal-ads. They see it as a chance to put all their favorite healthy ingredients in one meal. They will order a salad as a main course.

- Thin people prefer a salad over pasta because they feel better in their bodies after eating.

- Thin people love to find ways to add more veg-etables and greens to their daily diet.

- Thin people focus on the nutrients, fiber and vitamins a salad can provide.

Food in the Fridge

- Cut-up fresh veggies that are ready to go with some low-fat dressing or dip make a great easy snack.

- Cut up lemon, lime, and other fruit to spice up your water. Keep them next to a pitcher of water in the fridge.

- Have veggies on hand for salads and fruit for snacks. The more colorful fruits and veggies you have, the more they will stand out when you open the fridge.

- Include plenty of protein choices for dinner: eggs, meat, and fish to start.

15

BRAIN/BODY CONNECTION
The brain connects the body and mind—the key to targeting resides in the brain

Your brain controls your body. On these pages we will focus on how your brain can work specifically to help you with exercise.

Your brain is constantly sending signals to your body without you being aware of it. Many of your body's functions are automatic and happen whether or not you think about

them. When it comes to moving your muscles, your brain has created what is called "motor patterns," which are a series of motions you make often. The muscles you use in your already established motor patterns have a solid and strong connection to your brain. If you target a muscle that you already use, it's likely that the muscle is "used to" moving in a certain way.

Spark Plug

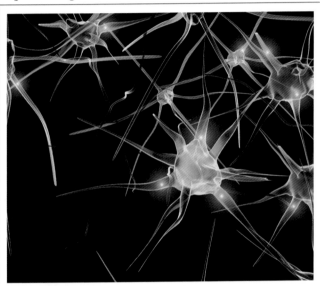

- Your brain connects to your muscles through an electrical impulse that travels from your brain to the nerve ending that stimulates the muscle.

- The bigger the "charge," the more muscle you will engage.

- Being more clear in your mind about what muscles you want to move can direct the charge to the right places.

- There are many chemical and electrical reactions that happen from brain to muscle movement.

Flipping a Switch

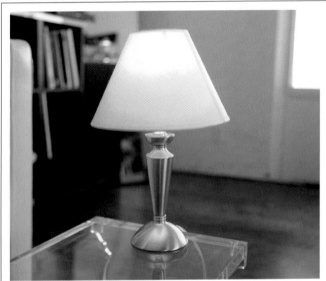

- When you flip the switch on a lamp, you do not need to think about whether or not the lamp will turn on.

- When you move without thinking, your body naturally engages the muscles that have performed these motions before. It's automatic.

- Thinking about and becoming aware of your body and what you want it to do can take you to a whole new level of engaging and controlling your muscles.

16

Adding new exercises and a stronger focus with your mind can actually activate more muscle fibers within that muscle and use parts of it that have not been used before. Just by adding more focus, you can stimulate greater results from that muscle.

Incorporating new exercises can create new motor patterns and help you use muscles that you do not commonly activate. All of this brain activity results in more muscle activity and can dramatically increase your results. People often say, "I felt muscles I didn't even know I had," but the truth is that when we use our muscles in the same way over and over again, those muscle fibers become strong and usually do most of the work. Adding a few new exercises and different ways of using your body will activate dormant fibers in the muscles you are already using. This may result in a new "soreness" you have not felt before. These new ways of movement will either activate new muscle fibers or new muscles!

A Guided Path

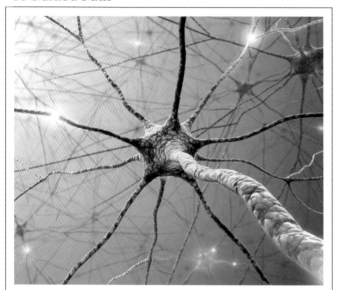

- Like a mousetrap or hiking trail, the movements you have already learned to do become embedded in your mind and muscles.

- When you learn a new sport or skill, you often feel uneasy or unsure at first on how to move your body.

- The more you practice a new motion, the more you will create another trail or new path from the brain to the muscle.

- Learning new movements activates more muscle. Change it up or learn something new every few months.

Basics of the Mind-Body Connection

- Becoming aware of your body can help you to maximize the use of all your muscles.

- Using visualization to connect your brain to the parts of your body you want to work can increase your ability to turn on those muscles.

- Learning a new skill or exercise may feel awkward at first because your mind has not created a motor pattern yet.

- Learning new sports, skills, and exercises helps you to utilize more of your body.

ISOMETRIC AB CONTRACTIONS

You can get an ab workout all day long with these "invisible" contractions

There are three types of muscle contractions: concentric, eccentric, and isometric. Concentric contractions occur when a muscle gets shorter, or "smaller," which happens when the two places it's connected are moved together. Imagine a biceps curl: When you bend your elbow and lift the weight, your biceps get smaller and "fuller" because it is

concentrically contracting. Eccentric is the lengthening of a muscle from a contracted position back to the attached length. Now imagine lowering the weight back down from that end range of motion for the biceps curl. The biceps was shorter and contracted and now it's lengthening as you extend your arm back down. Isometric is a contraction that

Isometric Abs at a Desk

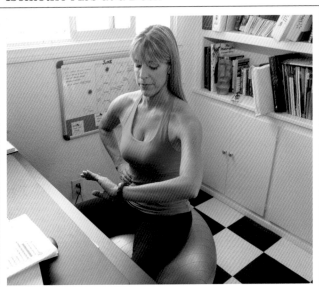

- Sit in an upright posture, feet flat on the ground, back off the chair with your shoulders down and back.

- Draw in the belly button and pull it close to your back without moving your rib cage or pelvis.

- Imagine that you could bring both sides of your rib cage closer together to meet in the middle. Do not forget to breathe. Hold this contraction for 30 to 60 seconds, squeezing with a moderate to intense effort.

Isometric Abs while Driving

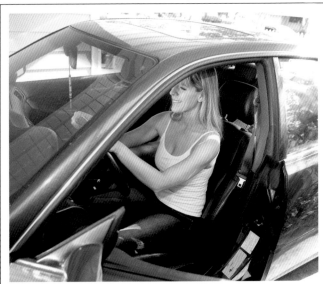

- Using all the same cues as you did seated at your desk, you can create an ab exercise while driving, too!

- Make sure for safety that you are able to do this exercise with ease without getting distracted from driving.

- You can "squeeze to the beat" and use your music to help you hold the contraction longer.

- Isometric abs can be done anytime, anywhere—it just requires some focus.

does not move—it's a holding of the muscle in the same amount of contraction so that it stays the same length.

Your abs connect your rib cage to your pelvis. You can do a simple isometric abdominal exercise all day long by imagining that you are pulling your rib cage closer to your pelvis without moving. Because your brain is now talking to the muscle, it will engage. Learning how to isometrically contract your abs can help you create core exercises that you can do while sitting at your desk or even while driving!

Most people think that in order to contract or use a muscle they have to move it. I often ask clients to contract their abs and they bend their spine or tilt their pelvis. These are examples of concentric contractions. What I want you to learn is that you can contract your abs (and every other muscle) with your brain and not by moving! No one needs to know that you're doing the exercise. You can turn on the muscles; they can contract and feel tighter without you moving your body. This is the basis of isometric contractions.

Isometric Squat

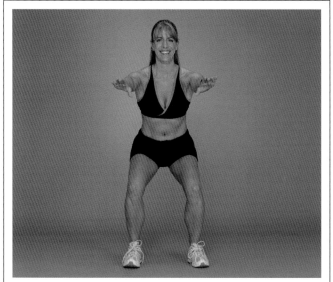

- You can create an isometric exercise from any exercise you currently do.

- The most common for the lower body is the wall sit or isometric squat.

- Because we all fold and bend differently, first find the right squat form for your body. You may need to use a ball against a wall.

- With your feet flat and weight evenly distributed, squat with about 20 percent of your full range of motion first to test it out.

Plank

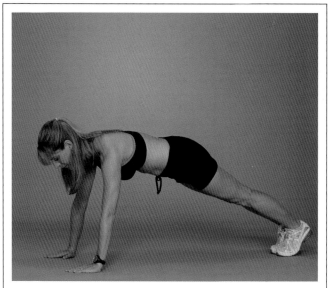

- The most common upper body isometric exercise is the plank, which is like a push-up, but you hold the starting position instead of bending and straightening your arms.

- Hands should be no wider than shoulder width apart, feet together, and back at the same height as your head.

- Keep abs engaged to protect your back. Imagine pushing away from the floor as you hold the position.

- Start with 3 sets, holding for 30 seconds.

THE MIND PLAN

What tools will you use to train your brain while you train your body?

Now that you understand the power of your mind, have an awareness of your "Exercise Story," and have some tools to choose from to help reprogram your mind, what will you do? Creating a plan for your mind is like creating a plan for your body. It will require a little preparation and planning to get started and then a commitment of using the tools you choose.

If this is all new for you, you may want to simply start with

keeping a journal. Having an outlet to express what is in your mind is often very effective in being able to clear your mind of your daily clutter. If you can clear you mind of that daily clutter, you leave space to fill it with more positive, supportive thoughts and beliefs. Journaling can be as simple as spending 5 minutes before you go to bed to write down how you feel, why, and acknowledge some of the positive parts of the day. You don't want your journaling to be mostly negative, so

Start a Journal

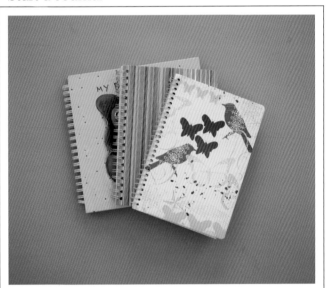

- A journal can be a precious reflection of your thoughts and emotions.

- Journaling provides a safe outlet for you to "unload" your thoughts and feelings without confrontation or consequence.

- You can choose a free form style of writing what comes to you or using a predesigned journal that guides you with questions to answer and things to focus on.

- Journaling can take 5 minutes before bed or can be used as a therapeutic tool.

Try a Guided Journal

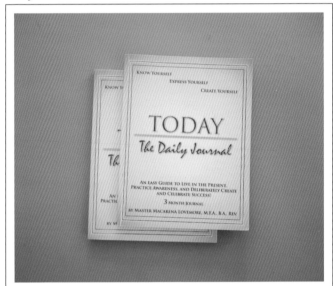

- If you have never journaled before but would like to begin, I would suggest using a guided journal to get you started.

- A blank page can sometimes intimidate people. Using a guided journal allows you to write short phrases or sentences

- instead of paragraphs.

- I like to use the Daily Journal at night before bed to clear my mind, reinforce what went well, and to focus on gratitude.

- This prepares me to open my mind to hypnosis audios so they are more effective.

make sure to end on a positive note.

After you have cleaned out your mind, you may choose to do hypnosis before or as you go to sleep. Because you will most likely fall asleep, this whole mind program should only take you 10 to 15 minutes of conscious awake time. Can you make 15 minutes available before bed each night? Think about what you are willing to do, what is easiest, and start there. You can also add more tools and time later when you see the effects taking place and want to invest more time.

Use Hypnosis CDs

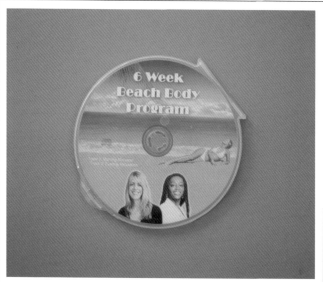

- Hypnosis CDs are easy to use, can be used for many years, and cover all kinds of issues and concerns.

- My 6 Week Beach Body Program has twelve different creative visualizations that focus on exercise, eating, cravings, motivation, and relaxation.

- There are other programs out there that deal with happiness, wealth, relationships, success, and more.

- The key to using hypnosis audios is repetition and immersion. You are introducing a new way of thinking—the more you practice, the better you get it!

Why Your Mind Matters

- The mind is the most important aspect of creating a healthy lifestyle change.

- The use of "willpower" will always fail, because your subconscious programmed beliefs will always be stronger.

- Changing your core beliefs will make lifestyle changes, weight loss, eating habits, and exercising easier and enjoyable!

21

GADGETS

Magic machines that promise amazing results in no time

You have seen the infomercials and ads for machines that claim you only need to do 5 minutes of exercise a day for amazing results. The problem with these claims is in the fine print that you don't read until after you have purchased the product! Your mother was right: If it seems too good to be true, it just might be. If you are an overweight, out-of-shape, sedentary person who believes that you really only need 5 minutes a day to look like the model on the show, you will be

sadly disappointed and frustrated—and you probably have a collection of these gadgets in your living room or garage.

This is not to say that the machines themselves are not usable or have some benefit—they might. But I encourage you to carefully read this book, follow the steps, and have some patience with this lifestyle change. It did not take you 30 days to get where you are, so it will probably take you more than 30 days to start to see results. Anyone can change

Ab Rollers.

- People are often attracted to machines and gadgets like this because they offer neck support.

- The problem in a product offering neck support is that it can sometimes create a crutch for the body.

- The head can weigh up to 12 pounds, and the muscles in the neck are supposed to be able to lift the head. I would not rely too much on external support, for fear of creating an imbalance.

Ab Rollout and Wheels

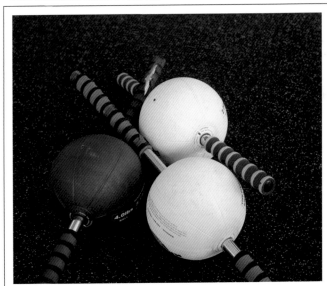

- Many ab products are wheels or balls that make it look easy and fun to work on your abs.

- While they may target abs differently than other exercises, they are generally very advanced for other muscles in your body.

- Work up to using these pieces more often, as they require arm and core strength.

- Do not rely on one machine to do it all. Your body adapts as it gets stronger and will need different exercises and intensity levels to progress.

his or her behavior for 1 to 3 months and experience results. The question remains whether or not you can keep those results forever.

Trampoline

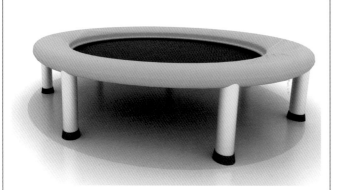

- Trampolines are not a one-stop shop. They will not produce dramatic weight loss and they do not target the upper body.

- A trampoline can be great to help lymph drainage and it's easier on joints.

- The fact is you bounce up and down, over and over, which will offer mainly cardio benefits.

- Depending on your fitness level when you start, this exercise can strengthen your ankles, spine, hips, and legs.

Ab Vibrating Belt

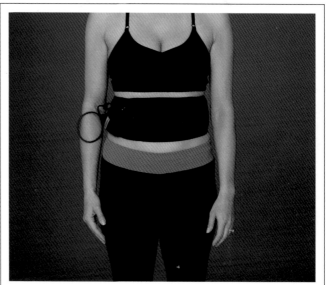

- There are belts on the market with claims that they can tighten your abs with the press of a button.

- Electrostim passively sends a signal to the muscle to contract, bypassing your brain.

- While electrostim may innervate your abs, the amount of stimulation is not enough to build significant muscle and will not burn many calories or reduce body fat.

- A belt may enhance your ab program but will not get you results if you don't exercise and eat properly.

STARVATION DIETS
Eating very few calories is not only dangerous but also kills your metabolism

Let's address some of the fad diets that have you reduce your calories so dramatically that you can't help but lose weight. A lot of them are 100 percent liquid based and actually are a form of starvation. When you stop eating, or eat an extremely low number of calories, you will lose weight. The key question is: Do you know where that weight comes from?

When you step on the scale, you are weighing your mass. Your mass consists of everything: skin, bones, blood, water, organs, hair, muscle, and fat. When you lose weight, it most likely is made up of one of three things: water, muscle, or fat.

Think of your body as a car. Your car will stall and stop when it runs out of gas, right? Your body will not stop if you don't

Muscle versus Fat

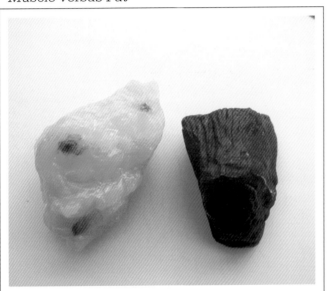

- People often say that muscle weighs more than fat which is not entirely true.

- Here is an example of 5 pounds of fat and muscle. As you can see, the 5 pounds of fat is larger than the muscle and takes up more room.

- Muscle is more dense than fat, so if we compare the same size of muscle to fat, the muscle would weigh more. But a pound is a pound.

- Muscle requires energy, so having more muscle increases your metabolism.

Lemon, Water, Cayenne, and Honey

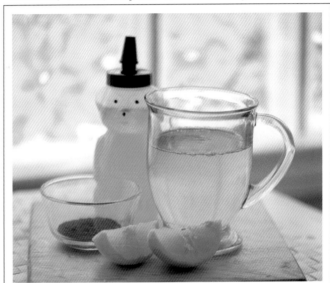

- One of the most common unhealthy detox diets consists of hot water, lemon, cayenne pepper, and honey.

- People drink this combination for days or even weeks with no food.

- Consuming a low-calorie

- protein-free drink as your only source of fuel is basically a starvation diet.

- Because the body is not getting enough nutrients to function day to day, your body will break down your muscle tissue to use as energy. Over time this will decrease your metabolism.

eat, but it will have to create energy and take it from somewhere else in the body in order to keep going once you have "run out of gas." The body will break down your muscle tissue and use it for energy before it will use fat stores. If your body is using its own muscle tissue as energy, your metabolism slows down, which makes it harder in the future to lose weight—and easier for you to gain it back. Your muscle makes up a large part of your overall metabolism so having more of it means you burn more calories naturally. Protecting and adding to your muscle mass is crucial for losing weight

and keeping it off. My simple advice is to work on eating a healthy and balanced diet that fits your life and goals. Eat three meals a day with one snack, and space out your meals every 4 to 5 hours. After 6 hours, your gas tank is on empty.

Hollywood Juice Diet

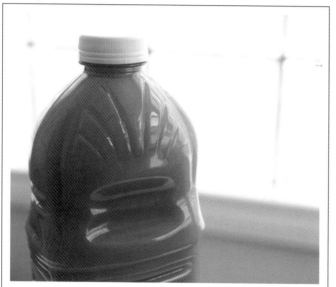

- There are many versions of liquid-only diets out, including the Hollywood diet or cabbage soup diet.

- Because of the lack of calories and nutrients, the body goes into "fight or flight" mode.

- In order to survive, your body will break itself down and use muscle tissue for energy.

- People who do these diets gain more weight back when they are finished than what they lost because they have lowered their metabolism.

Facts about Detox Diets

- Make sure you check the science behind detox diets and choose one that has ingredients to protect your muscle tissue.

- Any juice-only diet will compromise your metabolism, making it harder to lose weight later.

- Fasting is normally short-term; if used for weight loss, it will do more harm than good.

- Long-term success and optimal health come from balanced eating, not extreme restriction.

ONLY 6-MINUTE ABS?

A great place to start, but you'll need to incorporate cardio for real fat-burning results

We have already covered spot reducing, so you know that exercising only your abs will not necessarily "burn the fat" off your midsection. But how much time should you spend working on your abs? There is a formula we will cover later for creating a balanced exercise routine, but if your focus is abs, you will center the program on choosing exercises to build muscle, burn fat, and work your abs.

There are programs that promote 5- or 6-minute ab routines, and sometimes they do work. If it will work for you depends on how "in shape" and fit you are right now. For someone who is already athletic and lean, adding extra ab exercises will be the icing on the cake. If you are someone

Start Small

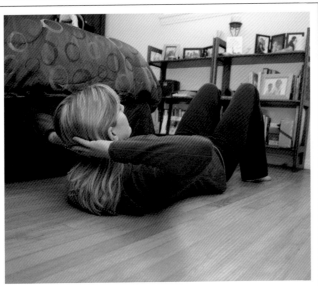

- Motivation and time are the biggest factors in getting started on any exercise routine.

- Start by doing 5 minutes a day when you get out of bed in the morning or before you go to sleep at night.

- Adding some small amount of exercise as part of your daily ritual will help you get excited to do more.

- You can feel and maybe even see some small changes by doing 5 minutes a day for 20 to 30 days.

Work Out During Commercials

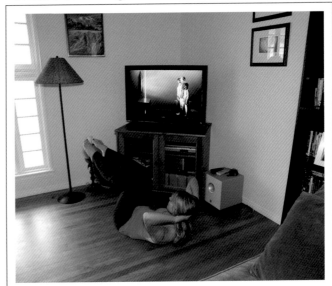

- Many people claim they do not have time for exercise, yet they have time for at least a 30-minute television program every day.

- Play a game with yourself to do some exercise during commercials. You are guaranteed to get at least 10 minutes of exercise during a 30-minute program.

- In 10 minutes you could do 3 sets of abs and 3 sets of legs. This would be a great start!

with 10 to 30 pounds or more to lose and have no muscle definition at all, doing an abs-only routine will not get you where you want to be anytime soon.

To achieve your goals, you will want to focus on diet, cardio, and exercising other muscle groups, but you can get started now by spending a little time strengthening your abs, which will prepare your body for harder and longer durations later. If you decide to add 5 to 10 minutes of abs now, adjust your expectations for feeling tighter and stronger. Don't step on the scale, hoping for massive weight loss.

Some people report feeling more motivated to follow better eating habits or do more cardio when they consistently add a minimum of 5 to 10 minutes of ab exercises. Because you can "feel the burn," that physical sensation is a reminder to stick to your plan. Do what is best for you, but know that 5 or 6 minutes of ab-only work is not enough for a beginner exerciser to achieve dramatic results.

Try a DVD

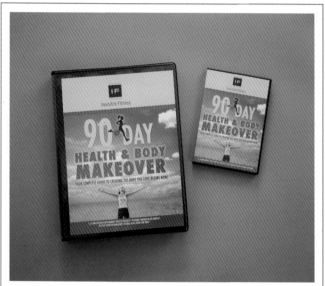

- Many of us already have a DVD—or ten—around that could help us start exercising.

- If you are feeling unmotivated to create your own exercise routine, stick in a DVD you already own.

- Check out the Invisible Fitness 90-Day DVD for exercises you can do anywhere.

- Use what DVDs you have and rotate them to get started. A DVD can be a great tool at least temporarily!

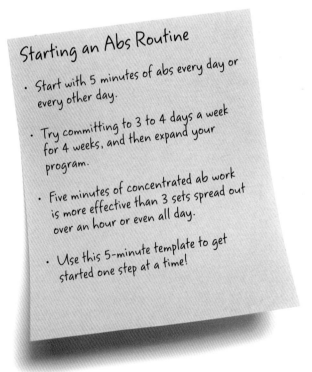

Starting an Abs Routine

- Start with 5 minutes of abs every day or every other day.

- Try committing to 3 to 4 days a week for 4 weeks, and then expand your program.

- Five minutes of concentrated ab work is more effective than 3 sets spread out over an hour or even all day.

- Use this 5-minute template to get started one step at a time!

FAT FREE OR LOW FAT?
Which is best? You might be surprised to find out!

First I have to bust the myth on the word fattening. It is incorrect to call something fattening, because one food group does not necessarily always convert into adipose tissue, or fat, in the body. When you think of something that is fattening, you think of a food group or item that will cause you to gain excess body fat because you ate it. The body does not work like that.

All foods can be converted into fat, period. Fat as a macronutrient is important for your brain, which is more than 50 percent fat. Fat also supports the lining of organs and helps create cell membranes. It can also satiate you so you feel more full and satisfied with less food. So the bottom line is this: You need fat in your diet for a healthy body, functioning brain, and strong cell membranes and to feel satisfied with a meal.

Fat-free foods are mostly processed, chemically engineered

Fat Free = Sugar Full

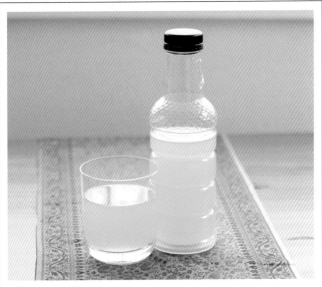

- Fat-free products often contain a high amount of sugar or additives.

- Sugar is fat free but can easily be stored as fat if the body does not need to use the energy it produces once it is digested.

- Sugar converts quickly into energy in the body and can more easily create adipose tissue than eating fat can, because it takes the body longer to break down fat.

Empty Carbs = Excess Calories

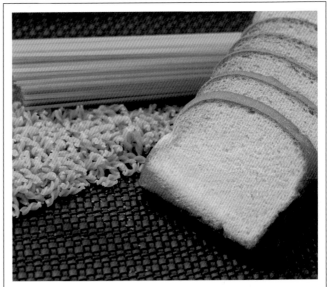

- Breads and pasta are relatively fat-free foods but are high in calories. Most breads and pastas are considered empty nutrition, because they offer no great health benefits.

- Breads and pastas are examples of fat-free foods that can easily help put fat

on your body because of their high calories and lack of nutrients.

- Consuming some fat, protein, and fiber along with these foods can help your body use them as energy all day long instead of storing them as fat.

foods that contain a high percentage of sugar and simple carbohydrates. Because of their high-sugar and carbohydrate content, they spike insulin levels and are more likely to turn into adipose tissue faster than their full-fat counterparts. Carbohydrates break down into glucose in the body. Imagine eating a scoop of fat-free sorbet on an empty stomach. Because all the calories come from simple sugar, the body is able to break this down easily and quickly. Once it's broken down, this energy is sent into the body to either be used as energy or stored as fat. Gaining fat from a fat-free item like sorbet will likely put pounds on faster than a moderate amount of good fat in every meal. When you are choosing your foods, make sure there is a small percentage from fat to help slow down absorption.

Fat-Free Cheese

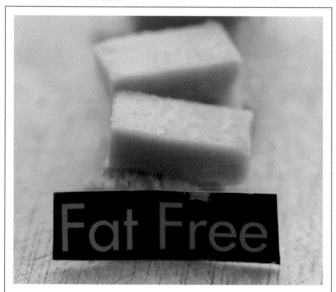

- Fat-free cheese often lacks taste and has extra preservatives and chemicals in it.

- Because fat-free cheese has no fat, the body breaks if down faster, just as it does carbohydrates.

- Low-fat cheese can offer a reduced amount of fat and calories while still offering flavor and integrity.

- Cheese has fat in it, and you need some fat in your diet. Enjoy a cheese that you love in moderation and limit those that have added preservatives.

Fat-Free Sweet Snacks

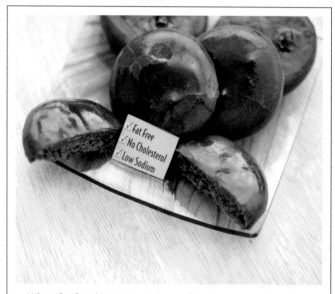

- When fat-free brownies and cookies came out, people ate them two and three at a time, because they were perceived as being the healthier choice.

- An average full-fat brownie has 190 calories, 9 grams of fat, and 14 grams of sugar. Compare that to two fat-free brownies, which have 110 calories and 22 grams of sugar each. That's 44 grams of sugar without any fat to slow down its breakdown—it's like an insulin injection!

- Our obsession with fat-free led to massive overeating and an increase of body fat.

THE CARB MYTH

Carbohydrates are not bad for you—it all depends on which ones you choose

Do you know what a carbohydrate is? Most people think of bread, pasta, rice, and starchy foods when they think of carbohydrates. This may be true, but the best carbohydrates for your body are actually fruits and vegetables, which many people don't realize are also carbohydrates.

Carbohydrates break down into glucose, and the body uses this sugar as its main energy source. Carbohydrates are needed to provide energy to the body like gas provides energy for your car. But unlike the old paradigm of the Food Guide Pyramid, we function best on large servings of vegetables with some fruit and very little starch.

Our DNA is not very different from that of our caveman

Vegetables

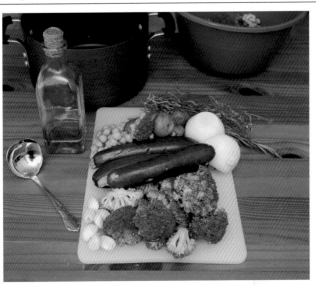

- People often only eat the same few vegetables over and over again. Make it a game to try a new vegetable each week!

- You can eat large volumes of vegetables without consuming a high number of calories.

- Vegetables contain fiber, which helps you to feel full, aids with digestion, and cleans you out.

- Americans lack proper fiber intake. Our caveman ancestors got 40 or more grams a day, while we struggle to get 20 grams.

Fruits

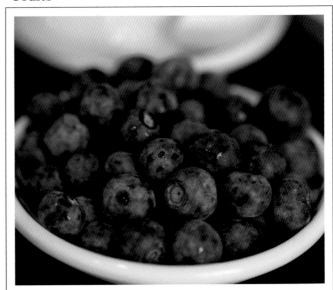

- Even though fruit has sugar, it's natural sugar. Fruit is nature's dessert.

- The most common fruits are apples, oranges, bananas, strawberries, peaches, pears, and blueberries.

- Other fruits we tend to forget include nectarines, apricots, blackberries, papaya, pineapple, melon, plums, raspberries, cranberries, grapefruit, tangerines, kiwi, watermelon, lemons, limes, guava, and mango.

- There are fruits for all seasons and climates. It's fun to try and incorporate something new on a daily basis.

ancestors who did not have access to processed foods and grains. We get our antioxidants and many vitamins from our vegetables and fruits. Our starches have to be fortified, because they naturally have less nutritional value in comparison.

I suggest eating the color of the rainbow in vegetables and fruits every day and limit starch intake to once a day, especially if you are on a weight-loss program. Vegetables and fruits are mostly water, so you can eat large quantities, especially vegetables, and not consume a high number of calories.

Quinoa

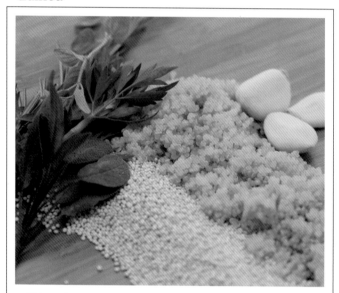

- This ancient grain is worth talking about because it's also a complete protein. It has all nine essential amino acids.

- Quinoa can be used in place of rice or couscous and is gluten free.

- Quinoa is loaded with the amino acid lysine, which is essential for tissue growth and repair. It is also a good source of manganese, magnesium, iron, copper, and phosphorus.

- Quinoa cooks similarly to rice; read the package for cooking instructions and recipe ideas.

Rice and Potatoes

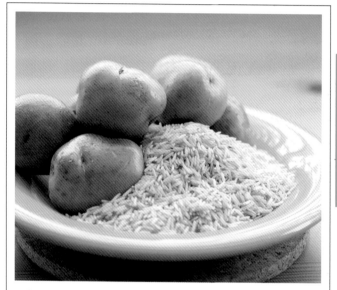

- Rice is a starch with nutritional value. It's high in an antioxidant called salicylic acid.

- Salicylic acid has been studied as a treatment for a variety of inflammatory bowel disorders and has been found to have a remarkable ability to prevent inflammation in the intestinal membranes.

- A potato is a healthful low-calorie, high-fiber food.

- Potatoes are a good source of vitamin C, vitamin B_6, copper, potassium, manganese, and dietary fiber.

THE MYTHS

31

FOOD SENSITIVITIES
Common foods may be keeping you fat by causing inflammation around your midsection

We know an allergy is a severe reaction to something. When it comes to food, it might manifest as blotchy, itchy skin; a swollen face or lips; or sneezing and congestion. Most people know instantly when they have an allergic reaction to a food. If you have symptoms, it might be a good idea to get tested for food allergies, but my guess is you already know if you have any food allergies if you try enough foods.

Food sensitivities are delayed reactions to certain foods. Food sensitivities cause inflammation over time and create "cravings" for certain foods. Odds are if you have strong cravings for something, you might be sensitive to it. The most common food sensitivities that often go undetected but

Corn

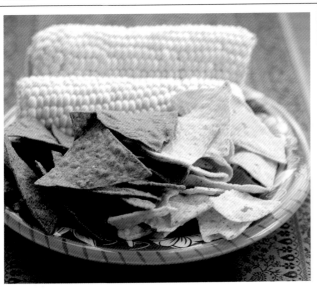

- Corn is a common cause of food sensitivity.

- Forms of corn include fresh, canned, creamed, frozen, tortillas, chips, oil, popped, cornmeal, and cornstarch.

- Corn can also be found in high-fructose corn syrup, baking powder, caramel color, dextrin, dextrose, fructose, maize, maltodextrins, sorbitol, and mannitol.

- For optimal nutrition, rotate your foods and consume corn just once a week to be safe.

Yeast

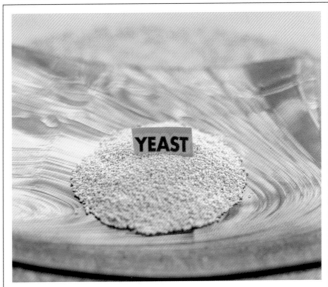

- Yeast is used in the fermentation of sugars, such as baker's yeast in bread production, brewer's yeast in beer fermentation, and yeast in wine fermentation.

- Yeast infection is extremely common.

- A yeast allergy is commonly known as candida.

- Yeast infection carries the widest spectrum of symptoms of any food sensitivity: skin problems like ringworm, gastrointestinal problems, lethargy, headache, breathing difficulties, and mood swings.

cause problems are gluten, corn, dairy, yeast, soy, and nuts. It is amazing to see what the body cannot digest properly due to lack of enzymes or overexposure.

Common side effects of having undetected food sensitivities include digestion issues, irritable bowel syndrome (IBS), weight gain, bloating, gas, chronic joint pain, weight-loss resistance, congestion, coughing, migraine headaches, chronic fatigue, attention deficit hyperactivity disorder (ADHD), eczema and other skin disorders, asthma and other respiratory problems, arthritis, and fibromyalgia.

Because food is the number one fuel we put into our bodies every day, it is a good idea to know the reaction your body has to the foods you eat. If you want a fit and firm core but always feel bloated and puffy around your middle, identifying and removing foods that you are sensitive to can make all the difference. Healing your gut and rotating your diet can help you to drop water weight and even body fat faster than you have experienced before. Is your food helping or hurting you? You can get tested for food sensitivities any time to see what foods may be affecting you. Visit http://alcat.com.

Nuts

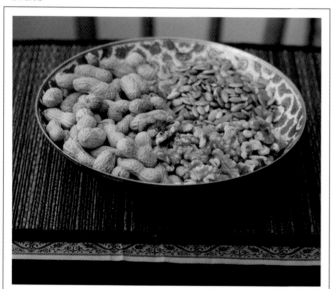

- Most people are familiar with nut allergies—a strong reaction to eating a nut that causes symptoms like hives or trouble breathing.

- Nuts are also one of the top five food sensitivities. Common side effects of food sensitivities include bloating, gas, and weight-loss resistance.

- Nut and nut oils are used in many foods, so be sure to read labels.

- Other common nuts that people often cannot digest properly are tree nuts, such as almonds, cashews, and walnuts.

Eliminate Certain Foods

- Getting tested is the best and fastest way to see how foods affect you.

- Try an elimination diet, where you remove one food at a time for 2 weeks then add it back in.

- Keep a journal while on your elimination diet so you know how your body reacts when you add foods back in. Then try removing another food and test the same way.

GLUTEN

This is not a fad but a common silent problem with weight-loss resistance

Gluten is the protein contained in wheat, barley, and rye. Many people are not able to break down this protein, so their bodies perceive the substance as a toxin. This can cause internal inflammation, which can result in digestive issues, bloating, weight gain, and more.

Besides wheat, barley, and rye, gluten is found in hidden places like the molds used to make chocolate candy, It's in the "caramel coloring" added to soft drinks, and it's in chewy candies, too. In cooking, gluten makes soups and gravies thicker and salad dressings creamier. It keeps yogurt and soft cheeses from getting runny, and dried spices from clumping. It's in the "natural flavoring," "modified food starch," and

Gluten-Free Bread

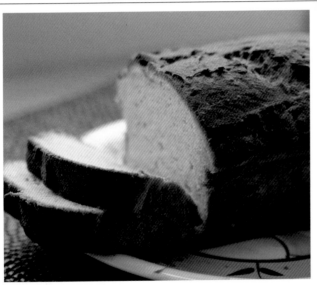

- The main fear people have about giving up gluten is giving up many of their favorite foods. But there is nothing that cannot be replaced with a gluten-free alternative to satisfy a craving or enjoy a treat.

- Gluten-free breads are made with alternative

flours, such as white rice, brown rice, tapioca, garbanzo bean, and arrowroot flour.

- Other gluten-free starches are amaranth; buckwheat; corn; flax; flours from nuts, beans, and seeds; millet; Scottish or Irish oats; potato starch; and quinoa.

Gluten-Free Pasta

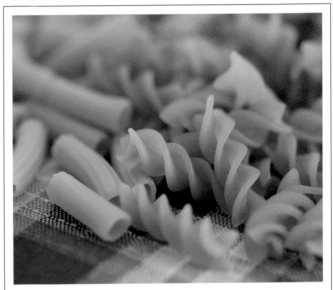

- I actually did not eat pasta until I became gluten free.

- Once I realized it was the gluten that was causing the bloating, I could occasionally enjoy some brown rice or quinoa pasta guilt free!

- From spaghetti to ziti, gluten-free pasta comes in all shapes and sizes.

- Replace your regular pasta with a gluten-free product, add your favorite sauce, and you might not be able to tell the difference!

"textured vegetable protein" added to thousands of food products. It's in veggie burgers, turkey burgers, and hot dogs, too. It's also used in the decaffeinating process for coffees and teas, and it's added to prepared mixed drinks, such as Bloody Mary mix, to lengthen the shelf life. Gluten is even used as a filler in medicines.

In July 2008, I tested a gluten-free diet for 14 days. After the first 10 days, I lost 4 pounds of water, which told me I had a sensitivity to gluten. I have been living a gluten-free lifestyle ever since. People have reported weight loss, alleviation of joint or back pain, repaired digestive issues, and more as a result of giving up gluten.

If you are sensitive to gluten, you could be holding on to several extra pounds of water and fat as a result of your body trying to "attack" this toxin. You may feel bloated all the time because of the inflammation. Trimming down your waist also means investigating other factors that could be causing issues for your digestion and water retention, including being sensitive to gluten.

Gluten-Free Baked Goods

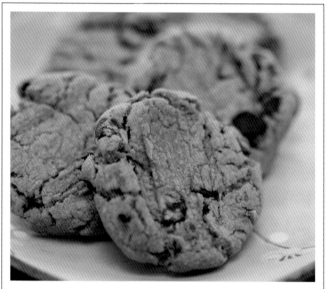

- We all like to have a treat now and then, especially for special occasions, holidays, and birthdays.

- My favorite chocolate cake is gluten free, and it's a huge hit everywhere I take it—no one knows the difference.

- Rich, sugary, starchy desserts should be eaten in moderation but should absolutely be enjoyed!

- You may need to experiment with finding the varieties that best fit your palate. Be patient—there are plenty of choices out there!

Gluten Substitutes

- Some foods are naturally gluten free: rice, potatoes, corn, quinoa, millet, and amaranth.

- Instead of toast with your eggs, have some potatoes. Switch out your couscous for quinoa.

- Rice is a gluten-free staple in Asian culture.

- If you are not sensitive to corn, it is a great substitute for wheat in Mexican cuisine. Italians cook polenta as a flavorful side dish.

DAIRY

Even if you have a sensitivity to dairy, you can enjoy cheese, yogurt, and ice cream

I have always said I would not give up my cheese—ever. But when I started to learn about food sensitivities, I got curious. I had to sit with the idea of being dairy free for a few months before getting tested, because I suspected that because I craved it and loved it so much, I must be sensitive to it. I was right! The good news with food sensitivities versus food allergies is that you can heal your gut and reintroduce those foods to your diet sooner rather than later.

Dairy sensitivity is probably one of the most undetected food sensitivities next to gluten. Because of this, there are many substitutes on the market to replace your favorite foods. Dairy is considered cow's, goat's, and sheep's milk

Cheese

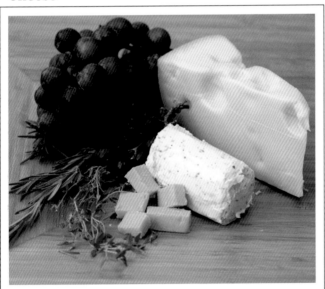

- If cheese is one of your favorite foods, don't worry, there are lots of replacements.

- Rice cheese is easy on the digestive system and comes in many flavors. Personally, I like cheddar best.

- Soy cheese is the most common replacement for dairy and can be found in most grocery stores.

- Daiya is a new cheese on the market that is soy and dairy free. Health-conscious restaurants and pizza places all over the country offer it as a dairy-free alternative.

Milk

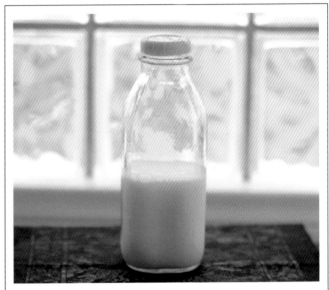

- There are several options for milk alternatives on the market.

- Rice, soy, almond, and coconut are the most common milk replacements.

- Regular milk has at least 5 to 9 grams of protein per 8 ounces. These alternatives

- do not have the same protein content. If you use milk substitutes, you will need to get your protein from other sources.

- If you drink milk for calcium, these sources do not provide ample amounts. You should get your calcium from other foods.

and can commonly be found in cheese, butter, milk, yogurt, and ice cream. Beyond the obvious foods that contain dairy, many other products contain dairy in the form of lactose or milk proteins. An example is a dairy protein called casein found in certain brands of tuna fish and alternative cheese products. Dairy and casein can also be found in packaged lunch meats, mayonnaise, potato chips, margarine, nondairy creamers, nondairy whipped topping, and products labeled lactose free.

Many people are sensitive to milk products because their bodies lack the enzyme called lactase. This enzyme, found in the gastrointestinal tract, is critical to the digestion of lactose. If lactase is missing or depleted, the gastrointestinal tract cannot adequately break down dairy and lactose.

Common symptoms of dairy sensitivity include stomach cramps, intestinal bloating or "pot belly," flatulence, diarrhea, headaches, and nausea. Most of us think these are common bodily functions, but they are actually your body exhibiting issues with digestion. I have found new and interesting alternatives to dairy!

Yogurt and Kefir

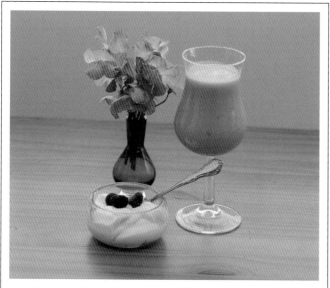

- Kefir is a probiotic form of milk, which means it has fermented and can actually help digestion.

- Going dairy free, I wanted to find a kefir substitute. I found coconut kefir.

- The main nutritional difference is that alternative dairy choices often lack protein. If you eat yogurt as a protein source, you will not find it here.

- Coconut yogurt makes a nice snack or dessert with some fruit.

Ice Cream

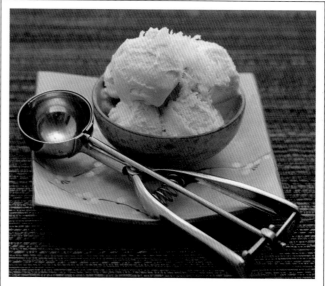

- With all the available flavors and brands of regular ice cream, you may be shocked that there are not many dairy-free alternatives.

- I have seen and tasted soy ice cream, rice ice cream, and coconut ice cream, and so far I like them all.

- Considering the high-sugar and low-protein content of these alternatives, eat them in moderation and after a meal with a significant amount of protein in it.

- Use some of your favorite toppings and enjoy a dairy-free sundae!

SUGAR

This sweet treat causes a host of problems when you ingest too much of it

There is not enough room in this chapter to list all the reasons why sugar is not good for you. Just like anything in life, everything in moderation is the key. But most people eat way more sugar than their bodies can handle. Here are a few things that excess sugar can cause: a suppressed immune system and impaired defenses against infectious diseases;

a rapid rise of adrenaline, hyperactivity, anxiety, difficulty concentrating, and crankiness; a significant rise in total cholesterol, triglycerides, and bad cholesterol and a decrease in good cholesterol; problems with the gastrointestinal tract, including an acidic digestive tract, indigestion, malabsorption, increased risk of Crohn's disease, and ulcerative colitis.

Soda

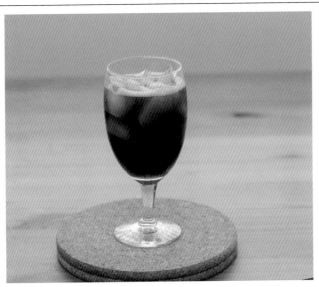

- Sodas are the single largest source of calories in the American diet, according to a report by the nonprofit Center for Science in the Public Interest (CSPI).

- Soda has been linked with obesity and type 2 diabetes because it contains massive amounts of sugar and calories. Consumption of soda can lead to increased insulin production, which can cause type 2 diabetes.

- Diet soda can cause food cravings because of the intensity of the sweetness from the chemicals that make up fake sugars.

Artificial Sweeteners

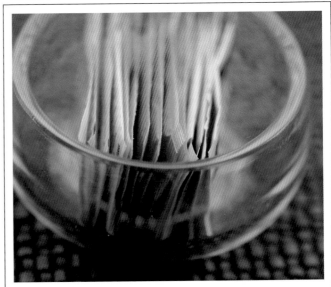

- The five FDA-approved nonnutritive sweeteners are saccharin, aspartame, acesulfame potassium, sucralose, and neotame.

- Artificial sweeteners are anywhere from thirty to seven hundred times sweeter than table sugar.

- Consuming large quantities of aspartame has been linked with symptoms such as headache, dizziness, mood swings, vomiting or nausea, abdominal pain and cramps, vision changes, diarrhea, seizures/convulsions, memory loss, and fatigue.

Sugar can also cause tooth decay and periodontal disease, and it of course contributes to obesity and diabetes.

In the last twenty years, we have increased sugar consumption in the United States from 26 pounds to 135 pounds of sugar per person per year! The average American consumes an average of 2 to 3 pounds each week, which is approximately 1,733 calories in sugar alone. Prior to the turn of this century (1887 to 1890), the average consumption was only 5 pounds per person per year!

Fast weight loss tip: decrease your sugar intake.

High-Fructose Corn Syrup

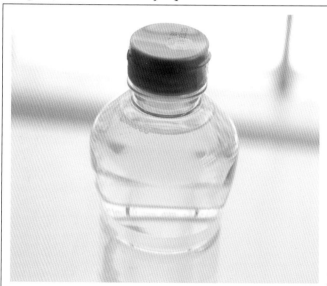

- High-fructose corn syrup extends the shelf life of processed foods and is cheaper than sugar.

- According to Princeton University a study of rats that consumed lots of high-fructose corn syrup showed that they became obese as a result.

- Posted on the university's website: "Rats with access to high-fructose corn syrup gained significantly more weight than those with access to table sugar, even when their overall caloric intake was the same."

Honey

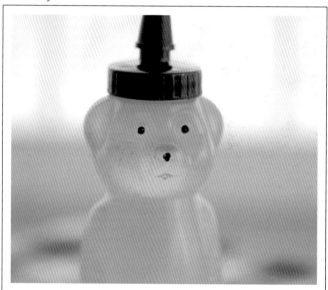

- Raw honey is an antibacterial, antiviral, and antifungal substance.

- It contains small amounts of the same resins found in propolis, which has been shown to possess cancer-preventing and antitumor properties.

- Honey contains a large amount of friendly bacteria, which may explain many of its therapeutic properties. It boosts immunity and can help with high cholesterol and type 2 diabetes because it can regulate blood sugar.

FOOD & NUTRITION

PROTEIN CHOICES
Eating the way we were designed to eat

Our DNA is not all that different from that of our caveman ancestors, who ate mostly meat and vegetables along with a few nuts and fruits when they were available. I do not recommend a "high-protein diet," as some of the more popular "carb-hating" diets out there do, as these actually can lower your metabolism. Instead I encourage my clients to consume protein at every meal.

Protein breaks down into amino acids, which help our bodies build and repair tissues. Protein takes longer than carbohydrates to break down in the body, so it provides energy longer than carbohydrates alone.

The average person does not eat enough protein. How much should you eat? Divide your ideal body weight in half. That is how many grams of protein you should aim to eat each day. For example, if your ideal body weight is 150 pounds, your goal should be to consume 75 grams or more

Meat

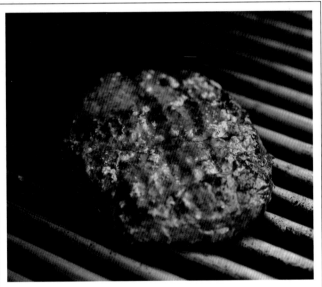

- When possible, choose grass-fed, free-range meats that are hormone and steroid free.

- Chicken, beef, pork, lamb, turkey, buffalo, and bison are good examples of animal proteins.

- Read labels to know what is in your meat. Ninety-eight percent fat free is based on volume not calories. Grass-fed meats are high in conjugated linoleic acids (CLAs), which have been shown to help increase muscle mass and help with weight management.

Eggs

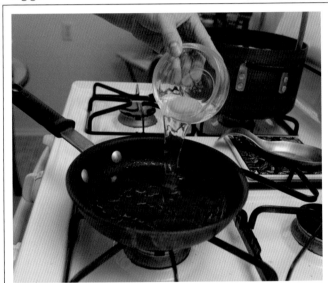

- Eggs are so versatile and can be eaten easily at any time of the day.

- They are a great way to consume a good amount of protein. And they can be prepared in many ways, from quiche, frittatas, egg bakes, egg salad, and deviled eggs, to scrambled, sunny-side up, and hard-boiled.

- One medium egg has about 65 calories, 4 grams of fat, and 6 grams of protein.

- One large egg white has 15 calories and 4 grams of protein.

each day. To ensure you get enough protein, center each meal around a protein choice. Increasing your protein can also help you burn more calories. Because breaking down protein has a metabolic effect on the body, eating more can actually help your body use more energy to digest it, resulting in a higher metabolism and possible weight loss.

When you concentrate on your protein choice for each meal, you decrease the amount of empty carbohydrates and calories you consume, which can also help speed up your weight-loss results. I encourage you to sit down and plan some meals around your favorite protein choices first and then add in a new one every 2 weeks. Make it a game to explore the farmers' market or grocery store with the perspective of trying some new foods you've never had before. You may discover a few new favorites!

Fish

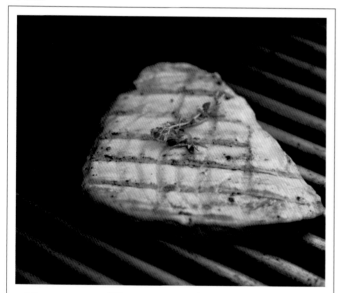

- There are many different varieties of fish such as bass, lobster, cod, flounder, and mahi-mahi.

- My new favorite snacks are canned sardines and oysters in olive oil. They do not need refrigeration and have up to 20 grams of protein and healthy doses of omega-3 fatty acids.

- Sardines and oysters are also low mercury options for those concerned about mercury toxicity.

- Fish in moderation can be great for your heart, brain, and skin and can be a tasty protein meal.

Soy

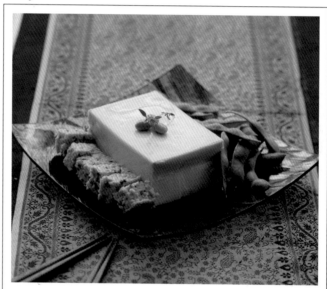

- Soy in its natural form is a great protein source, especially for vegetarians.

- Soybeans (edamame), tofu, and tempeh are great soy options to consume as protein substitutes.

- Denatured soy, such as soy protein concentrate, soy protein isolate, and soy used in fake meats and burgers, is not healthy for you. Soy has also been linked to elevated levels of estrogen, so use it sparingly and stick to the most natural forms.

CARBS & FIBER

Your mother was on to something when she wanted you to eat your vegetables

We do not eat enough fiber, period. I have heard that fiber is like a scrub brush that cleans out your body. There are two major kinds of fiber: soluble and insoluble. Soluble fiber dissolves in water to form a gel-like substance and helps to slow down the absorption of sugar into the body. Sources include oats, legumes (beans, peas, and soybeans), apples, berries,

vegetables, bananas, barley, and psyllium. Insoluble fiber facilitates the movement of material through your digestive tract and increases stool bulk. Sources include whole wheat foods, nuts, seeds, bran, and fruits and vegetables.

On food labels fiber is listed with the carbohydrates. Consuming fiber helps slow down the digestion of foods and

High-Fiber Vegetables

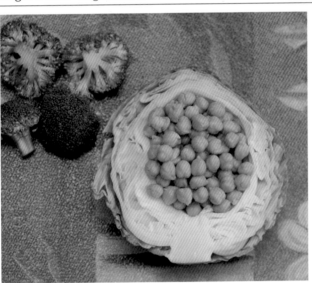

- The Food Guide Pyramid recommends that adults consume 25 grams of fiber each day. Our caveman ancestors got 40 to 100 grams a day. They did not have heart disease.

- Rather than taking a fiber supplement, try to get your daily intake of at least

  35–40 grams from food.

- Good sources include broccoli, brussels sprouts, cabbage, carrots, garbanzo beans, black beans, eggplant, kale, and lima beans.

- You will feel more satisfied with fewer calories when you increase your fiber.

High-Fiber Fruits

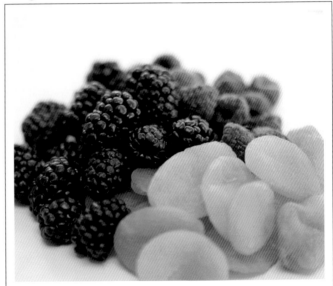

- Get some of your fiber from fruits, which are sweet and rewarding in many ways. Fruits with fiber are an easy way to increase your children's daily fiber, too.

- Try avocados, persimmons, apples, passion fruit, figs, dates, apricots, and blackberries.

- Eating more fiber keeps your digestive system happy and healthy.

- Baking with fruit is a good way to get your fiber. Make a tasty high-fiber dessert like an apple, apricot, or blackberry crisp—a simple and easy treat that's good for you!

allows the body to provide a more steady stream of energy. Adding more fiber to your diet helps regulate blood sugars and keeps you feeling fuller longer. Fiber also plays a role in weight control and helps fight heart disease and diabetes.

The best sources of carbohydrates are vegetables and fruits. Not only do they contain fiber in their skins, but they are also loaded with vitamins and antioxidants, which keep you younger longer! They also boost your immune system. At least 30 to 40 percent of your daily intake of calories should come from plant-based carbohydrates.

A Few Recommended Vegetables

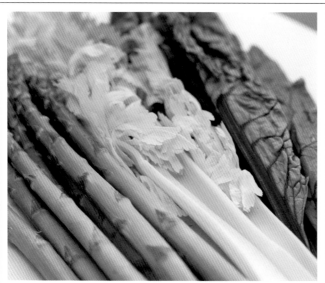

- You can add vegetables to every meal. Add some spinach, Swiss chard, or greens to your scrambled eggs in the morning.

- Have a salad for lunch or a lettuce wrap with beef, chicken, or turkey.

- Steam some veggies for dinner and try a new vegetable every week. Get your kids or family involved in making choices.

- Have some carrots, celery, or asparagus with hummus or dip as a snack.

A Few Recommended Fruits

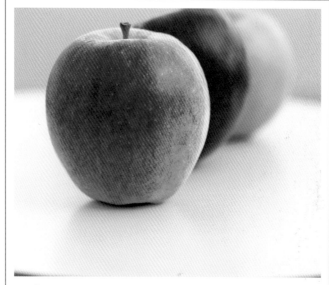

- When you start to decrease your refined sugar intake, fruit can be an excellent choice for that sweet treat.

- Eat all colors of fruits and alternate them to get the most vitamins and antioxidants you can.

- Fresh fruit with whipped cream, chocolate, or yogurt make a healthy and delicious dessert. Check to see what is in season and try to enjoy the best fruits all year round.

FOOD & NUTRITION

FAVORITE FATS
Feel full and satisfied and burn more fat!

Most of us love our fats, right? They do make our food taste good. But how much fat is too much? And does eating fat make you fat? We already covered the fact that dietary fat does not automatically turn into body fat. Dietary fats are essential to give your body energy and to support cell growth and help create cell membranes. They help protect your organs and your brain. Fats also help your body absorb nutrients, and they produce important hormones as well.

So fat is important, but how much should you consume? You will read many recommendations with different points of view on how much is the right amount. Low-fat diets, which fail to leave people feeling satisfied and offer less than optimal long-term success, are definitely not the way to go. Even if you have high cholesterol and heart problems, you still need healthy fats to help strengthen your cells so they can function optimally. Some popular very low-carb diets

Olive Oil

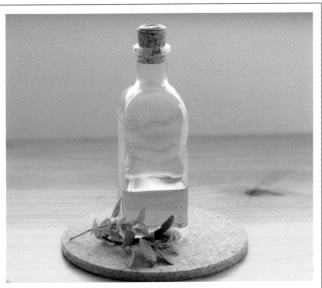

- Mediterranean diets include healthy amounts of olive oil. We know the people of this region have good skin.

- Olive oil has 5 milligrams of flavonoid polyphenols for every 10 grams of oil. These polyphenols are natural antioxidants that

can prevent heart disease, lower cholesterol and blood pressure, and reduce the overall effects of aging.

- Olive oil offers protection against heart disease by controlling LDL ("bad" cholesterol) levels while raising HDL ("good") cholesterol) levels.

Coconut

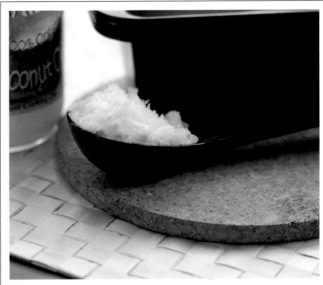

- Coconut is one of the healthier fats. It is my favorite fat by far.

- It offers many benefits. It keeps the skin, teeth, and hair healthy; helps with stress relief; maintains cholesterol levels and weight loss; boasts immunity; aids with proper digestion and

metabolism; strengthens the bones; and provides relief from kidney problems, heart diseases, high blood pressure, diabetes, HIV, and cancer.

- I cook and bake with coconut oil, and use coconut cream in place of dairy creamer.

recommend large amounts of saturated fats, which leave people thinner and with elevated LDL cholesterol levels—this is not good either.

I recommend that 25 to 30 percent of your diet should contain heart-healthy fat based on *The Paleo Diet* by Loren Cordain.

ZOOM

There are four major dietary fats: saturated, mono-unsaturated, polyunsaturated, and trans. The "bad" fats—saturated and trans—include refined oils, partially hydrogenated oils, shortening, and commercially deep-fried foods. The "good" fats—monounsaturated and polyunsaturated—come from fish, egg yolks, nuts, seeds, olives, durians, and unrefined oils. Read labels and investigate.

Avocado

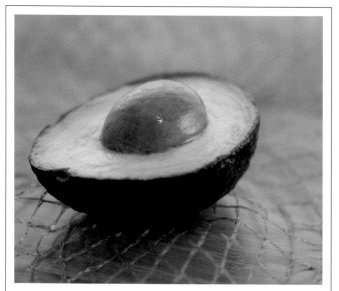

- Avocados provide nearly twenty essential nutrients, including fiber, potassium, vitamin E, B vitamins, and folic acid.

- Oleic acid in avocado can be used to lower blood cholesterol levels.

- Avocados act as a "nutri-ent booster" by enabling the body to absorb more fat-soluble nutrients, such as alpha- and beta-carotene and lutein.

- Add it to salads, eggs, and meats or make guacamole. You can even enjoy it alone with some tomato and pepper!

Nuts

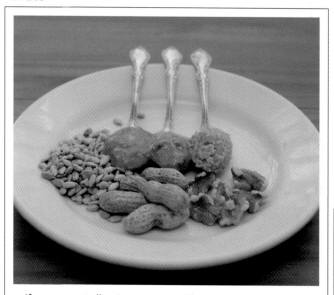

- If you are not allergic or sensitive to nuts, they are one of the best plant sources of protein with fat.

- They are rich in fiber, phyto-nutrients, and antioxidants such as vitamin E and selenium.

- There are many varieties to try and enjoy as a snack to keep blood sugar levels down and provide some protein and fat. There are so many nuts to choose from, you cannot get bored!

- My new favorite finds are walnut-cashew butter and sunflower butter.

YOUR SIX-PACK MUSCLE

The rectus abdominis—how it works and how to work it

The rectus abdominis is the muscle on the front of the body that's visible when someone is very lean. It is often referred to as the "six-pack." It connects the pelvis to the rib cage. When it contracts, it causes spinal flexion. One of the myths out there about the abs is that you have upper and lower abs. This probably came about because the rectus abdominis looks sectioned and because most people tend to focus on crunches, using their upper body as resistance, so they "feel"

the upper part of this muscle more than the lower part. But if you perform a reverse crunch or half crunch lower as I call it, you may "feel" the work happening closer to the pelvis in the lower part of the abdominals.

Because this muscle helps to connect the two halves of the body, upper and lower, it can be worked and moved in several ways. One option is to concentrate on and activate the fibers closest to your rib cage. You can contract or pull

Half Crunch Upper

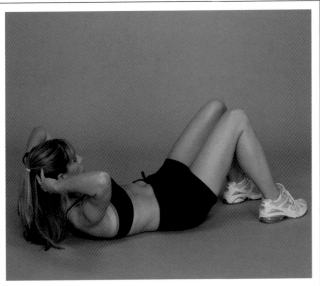

- This is the most common crunch. You lift only your upper body off the floor.

- People often feel the ab muscle fibers closest to their rib cage when doing this exercise.

- Even though you may feel it more in one half of your

abs, the entire muscle is working.

- The most common mistake to make with crunches is to pull with your head and neck, so be sure to keep them relaxed and focus on using your ab muscles.

Half Crunch Lower

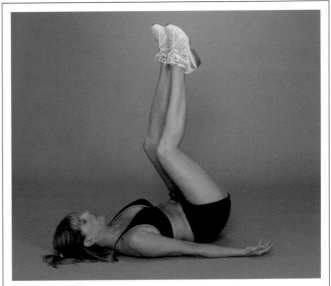

- Moving your lower body with your abs is usually much more difficult, because the lower body generally weighs more than the upper body.

- Because this is normally a very difficult exercise, start slow and expect it to be challenging.

- With your legs in the air, visualize your abs pulling your pelvis closer to your ribs.

- Use your ab muscles to lift your lower body, bringing it closer to your rib cage.

them closer to your pelvis to lift or move your upper body. Because of physics and mechanics, the weight of your upper body challenges the fibers closest to what is moving it. This is why you feel the "upper" part when you do a crunch. Another option is to focus on pulling your pelvis closer to your rib cage, using your lower body as resistance. This increases your awareness of the lower fibers of these muscles. The last option is to pull both sides into the middle—this is called a full crunch.

Even though the rectus abdominis is one of the first muscles you can see on your body because it is a surface muscle, it has many helpers beneath the surface to help move your body.

Full Crunch

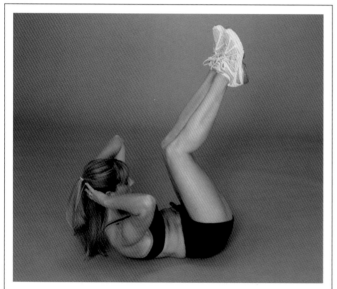

- Because the rectus abdominis connects the rib cage to the pelvis, we can move them independently or together.

- There are many variations of this exercise to make it easier or harder.

- Your form will depend on your structure.

- If you have long legs, you will get more movement in the lower half of your body than in the upper half.

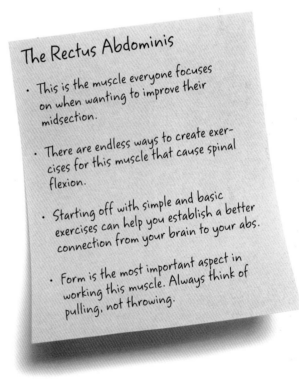

The Rectus Abdominis

- This is the muscle everyone focuses on when wanting to improve their midsection.

- There are endless ways to create exercises for this muscle that cause spinal flexion.

- Starting off with simple and basic exercises can help you establish a better connection from your brain to your abs.

- Form is the most important aspect in working this muscle. Always think of pulling, not throwing.

THE LOVE HANDLES

The external and internal obliques do more than hang over your jeans

The external and internal obliques are located in the area we often call "love handles," where our extra fat seems to hang on either side of our bodies. The obliques also connect the lower rib cage to the pelvis but have diagonal fibers and insert into the linea alba, which is the center line of the rectus abdominis that divides it into halves. Because the fibers run diagonally, they contract diagonally. These muscles help the rectus abdominis with spinal flexion and bending. They also act like springs that bring you back to center every time you walk or twist. All three of these muscles also provide stability for the spine.

I see a lot of people doing dangerous exercises in an effort

External Obliques

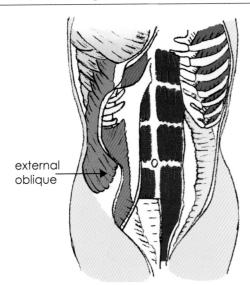

external oblique

- The fibers of the external obliques run downward.

- They attach the ribs to the pelvis in a diagonal direction.

- The external obliques help to stabilize and balance your motion when you walk.

- They allow the body to twist and rotate and also help with spinal flexion. Working them is important to keeping your active rotation strong.

Internal Obliques

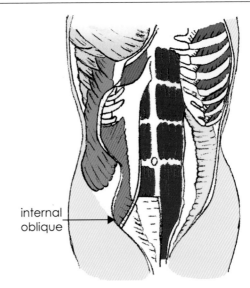

internal oblique

- These fibers run opposite and almost perpendicular to the external obliques.

- You cannot see these muscles on the surface but they are extremely important to keep you safe and strong.

- Always pay attention to your body and what it tells you. Soreness 24 to 48 hours after a workout is good as long as it is evenly distributed and goes away after 48 to 72 hours.

to target these muscles, but what people do not seem to realize is that they work all the time. The danger in using a lot of force in the positions that really emphasize the obliques is causing injury to the spine. Exercise should keep us stronger longer, not cause us to deteriorate faster. You can certainly do exercises to focus on the obliques, but know that these muscles always work with the rectus abdominis. Think of "pulling" the muscle together regardless of which one you are working and avoid fast movements and "throwing" your body.

Standing Rotation

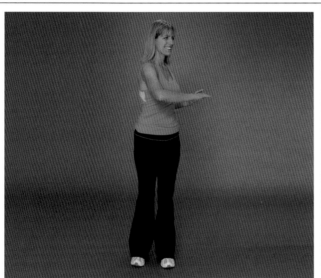

- To test your active range of motion, stand with your feet hip width apart.

- Without moving your feet, twist your upper body to the left as far as you comfortably can go. Pull yourself there slowly, do not throw or push.

- Test yourself to the right side as well and get to know what your body is capable of right now.

- As you get stronger and more flexible from the exercises in this book, you may increase your active range.

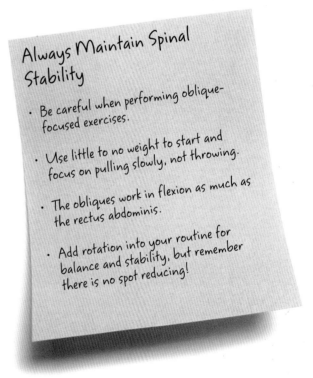

Always Maintain Spinal Stability

- Be careful when performing oblique-focused exercises.

- Use little to no weight to start and focus on pulling slowly, not throwing.

- The obliques work in flexion as much as the rectus abdominis.

- Add rotation into your routine for balance and stability, but remember there is no spot reducing!

KNOW YOUR BODY

A LAUGHING MUSCLE

The transversus abdominis can increase strength in all areas of your body

The deepest of all the core muscles is called the transversus abdominis. Its fibers run horizontally like a belt. When you cough or laugh, it activates and contracts by pulling in toward the spine. Some believe this is the most important core muscle because it is closest to the spine and can provide direct support of the spinal column. You cannot see this muscle when you look at someone's body, but it is important to be aware of its location so you can activate it with your mind instead of it simply being activated as a reflex when you laugh or cough!

The transversus is one of the muscles that act as your internal weight belt. When you consciously contract your

Bending Over = Bad Form

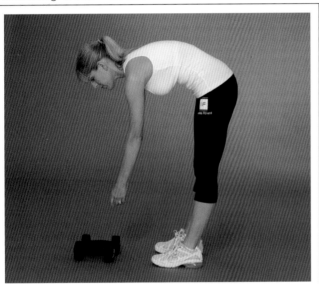

- Having a six-pack does not mean your abs automatically protect your back. You have to turn them on with your brain.

- A common posture used to pick things up is flexion at the spine, where the abs cannot really help you. In this position, your abs are not supporting you.

- All the resistance from your body and whatever you are picking up is being directed on the lower back and spine.

- Avoid this position when possible to protect your back.

Practicing Good Alignment

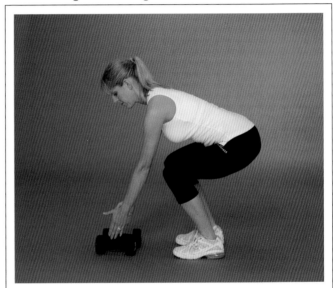

- With your spine upright and in alignment, you can now use your transversus abdominis and other ab and back muscles to support your spine.

- This position uses your legs more than your spine but gives you a greater strength advantage.

- Start by bending your knees and sitting back almost in a squat to start.

- Contract your transversus abdominis with your mind by pulling your belly button in toward your spine and squeeze.

50

transversus, you can actually increase strength production for all joints. Your abs, when contracted, pull everything into the center of your body, creating a foundation for other joints to move more securely.

I often say, and it's not a pleasant thought but a truthful one, that if you cut off your arms and legs, you can still live. This is because you were built from the inside out—middle first. Your core holds most of your major organs minus the brain and heart. Creating a strong core is not only about looking good, but also about performing better.

Test Your TVA

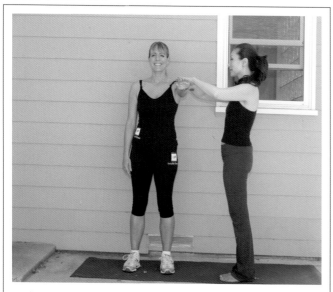

- This is a test you can do to help you understand the power of your core.

- With a partner helping you, stand with your stronger shoulder flexed in front of you, parallel to the floor.

- Have your partner push with both hands on your arm while you resist to test your shoulder strength.

- Concentrate only on the shoulder muscles as you resist. Notice your strength level.

Testing Position

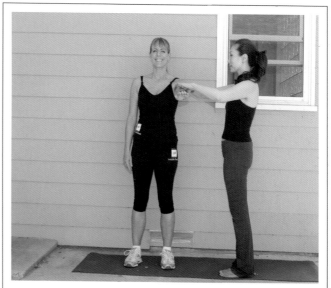

- Resume the position of holding the same arm out in front of you, shoulder flexed.

- This time pull your belly button in toward your spine and squeeze.

- Contract your abs as your partner pushes down on your arm to test your shoulder.

- Notice the difference in strength. You should have more when you use your abs.

LOWER BACK MUSCLE
Why the quadratus lumborum is so important for your abs

I like to think of this muscle as the "abs of the back." Most people only think about their lower back when they experience pain in that area. If you have no pain, you probably do not think about it much at all. If you have pain, you think about it often and treat this area with caution. First, I want to point out that lower back pain or discomfort does not necessarily have anything to do with this muscle. And if this muscle gets some exercise, it may feel sore just as any other muscle does.

One of the biggest myths about the lower back is that a weight belt can support your back. This is a myth because no external support can turn on muscle for you. If you want to protect your back, you have to use your muscles. Think about it this way: If I have a cast on my arm, it limits my range of motion, but I can still contract or relax the muscles inside. Too often people rely on weight belts to do their muscles' job of holding the spine tightly in good alignment. This can

Quadratus Lumborum

- The lower back muscle is called the quadratus lumborum (QL) and connects the rib cage to the pelvis.

- The QL acts like the abdominals but for the back.

- Most people feel tightness or stiffness here because of sitting all day.

- Soreness in this muscle is commonly mistaken for pain after exercise. If you feel a soreness or stiffness in your lower back after exercise, pay attention to see if it feels like muscle soreness. If you have pain, consult a doctor.

Bad Posture

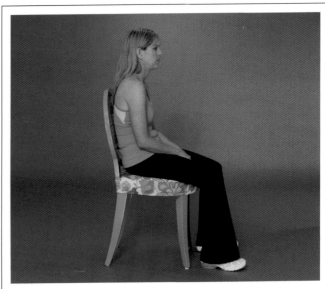

- Since most of us sit at our jobs, we likely do not hold a good posture all day long.

- The desk and chair support us either leaning back in the chair or forward on the desk.

- Your muscles are not working when you lean against something for support.

- Due to slouching and leaning, people often complain about back pain.

become dangerous when lifting heavy things, however, because it gives a false sense of security.

The bottom line: Your muscles are your internal weight belt. If you use them, you do not need anything else for support. Exercise them, keep them strong, and practice good posture and you'll never think you need a belt to do the work for you!

You can work the quadratus lumborum by doing a face-down spinal extension exercise. Lie facedown on the floor, lift your upper body off the floor, and then lower it back down to the ground and repeat.

Good Posture

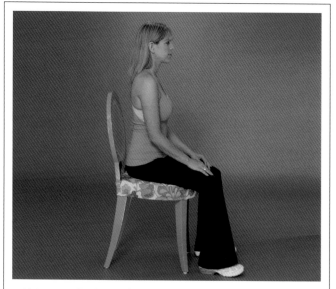

- Using your back muscles, you can hold yourself upright with your feet flat on the ground.

- This activation counts as low-level exercise for these muscles and will help you to strengthen them as well as burn more calories.

- You may have some soreness from doing this the first and second day. This will pass once you get stronger.

- If you are a beginner exerciser, try holding yourself up for 15 to 20 minutes to start and increase it by 10- or 15-minute increments.

Standing Posture

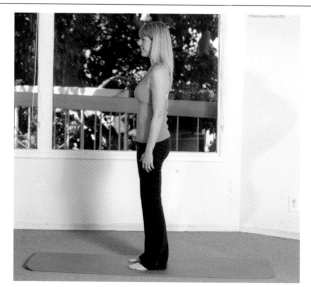

- Good posture is when your bones sit evenly on top of each other the way you were built.

- The chin should sit in a place so your ears are over your shoulders.

- Your shoulders should be down and slightly back with your rib cage floating over your pelvis.

- Your pelvis should be in neutral—not pushed forward or tucked in.

THE ABS SUPPORTER

Erector spinae—the little muscles with the big job of holding up your spine

A large and deep group of nine muscles make up the erector spinae, which helps support the spinal column and cause extension of the spine—also known as bending backwards. Strong erector spinae muscles can help with good posture and keep the back healthy and strong. It's important to know all your core muscles so that you can better connect with them when you exercise. The body is an amazing structure that was created with precision. Every muscle has a function and purpose, and you can better appreciate them and make wise choices about adding force based on this information.

When it comes to holding yourself upright in good posture, you first need to be aware of your posture and activate the

The Back Muscles

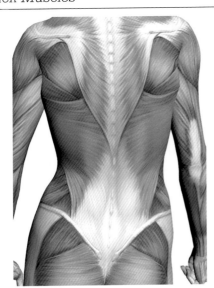

- There are many muscles that work at holding together the back. They range from large to small muscles connecting your bones from your head to your pelvis.

- Some you can see on the surface, like the latissimus dorsi and the trapezius.

- Others are under the surface, like the erector spinae muscles.

- Each one of these muscles has a specific job in moving or stabilizing the body. The body is an amazing, well-crafted structure!

The Erectors

- There are three main divisions of the erector spinae muscles: the spinalis division, longissimus division, and iliocostalis division.

- In each division there are three different muscles.

- They run from the back of the neck to the pelvis.

- They are the deepest "back" muscles you have and sit underneath the lats, trapezius, and rhomboids.

muscles with your brain. Once your muscles are activated, they need to be strong in order to continue holding you upright all day.

Many of my clients have said "make me stand up straight." This comes from a misconception about posture. Yes, you do need muscle strength and stamina especially if you are large breasted, pregnant, or carrying extra weight in the front of your body. But good posture starts in the mind first; it activates the muscles needed to make good posture happen. The more you consciously exercise these muscles, the more available they will be when you need them. Practicing good posture mean activating these muscles and others to hold your body in a upright position which often starts with chest up and shoulders back. Holding your body upright all day takes a lot of effort, so rest assured that your muscles are working hard to make that happen. Holding good posture all day can also increase the amount of calories you burn without you having to add exercise. It is exercise for these muscles to do their job!

Extending Your Spine

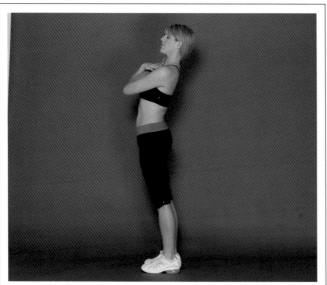

- Everyone has a different range of spinal extension.

- When you contract your spinal erectors, they pull your shoulders and spine closer to your lower back.

- Honor your active, pain-free range of motion and do not force excessive movement.

- Always contract these muscles slowly and imagine them pulling you backward.

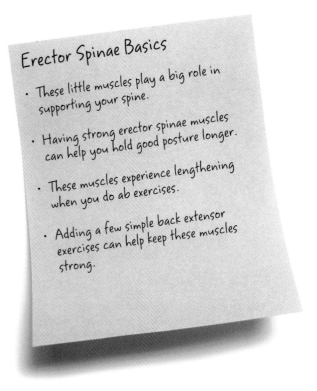

Erector Spinae Basics

- These little muscles play a big role in supporting your spine.

- Having strong erector spinae muscles can help you hold good posture longer.

- These muscles experience lengthening when you do ab exercises.

- Adding a few simple back extensor exercises can help keep these muscles strong.

55

MAT PILATES

Focused core training with Pilates can help you learn to control your core muscles

There are endless types of exercise programs and exercises you can do. We often get stuck repeating the same exercises over and over because they work initially. We like them, and so we trust that if we continue doing them, they will keep working. If you are bored with your basic ab exercises, trying something new like Pilates could make your workouts more interesting and help you to achieve greater results.

Pilates can be done in a class or privately, on a mat, or on a machine. This section will deal with the core work of Pilates, commonly called mat Pilates, which basically means that you don't use any equipment other than your body weight and a mat. Mat Pilates is a great way to use body weight resistance

Roll Up Start

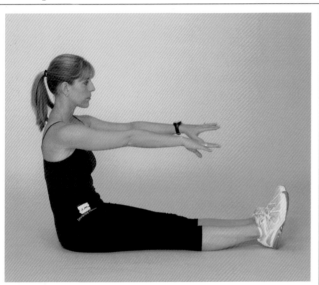

- Start seated, upright, with your spine tall and arms stretched out in front of you.

- You will begin by imagining that you are placing each vertebra on the ground one by one, starting with your pelvis and lower back.

- Tuck your pelvis and begin to slowly place your pelvis, then your lower back on the floor and work up your entire back.

- Keep your mouth open so you can breathe in both directions the entire time.

Roll Up Mid-range

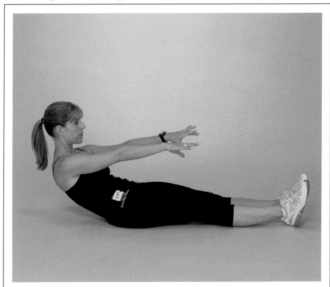

- Keeping your arms out as you lower to the ground will remind you to focus on small, precise movements of the spine.

- This is halfway down, but you can lower and place each vertebra on the mat one at a time all the way to your head.

- In reverse, you will lift from your head and neck first, and then pull each vertebra off the floor.

- Use your abs to control your speed and motion.

and control to challenge your body. Pilates mainly works on your core and will build abdominal strength, stamina, balance, and coordination. You also get some hip, glute, leg, and even arm work as well.

Pilates is not cardio work, but you can still work up a sweat. It's important to know what you gain from the exercises you choose, because all exercise is not created equal. Expect to achieve a stronger and maybe firmer core from the work you do in Pilates.

ZOOM

Pilates is very popular for people with back injuries and people who want to work on better posture, because all the exercises focus on the core first. As a beginner you can start with very little resistance and increase as you progress. If you are advanced, there are many variations for each exercise to make them harder and more appropriate for an advanced exerciser.

Inner Thigh Lift Start

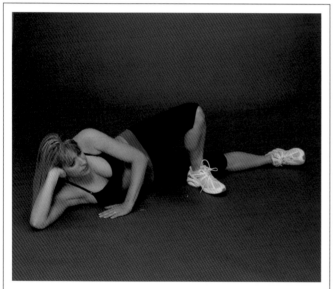

- Lie on your side and place your legs a few inches in front of you.

- Bring the foot of your top leg to the floor by bending your knee and bend the top leg over the bottom leg. Use your top hand to secure the top, bent leg.

- Make sure the leg is in neutral position and the side of your knee on the bottom leg is facing the ceiling.

- Rest your head on your hand or on the floor.

Inner Thigh Lift End

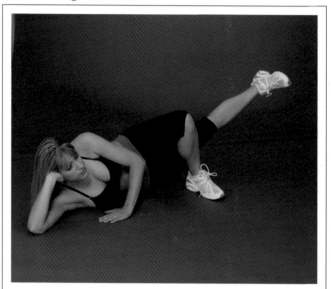

- Keeping the bottom leg straight, use your inner thigh to lift the leg as high as you can comfortably go.

- Keep your abs tight and imagine pulling your leg up with the muscles of your inner thigh.

- When lowering the leg, do not touch the floor and rest. Keep a slow pace up and down as you lift and lower.

- The weight of your leg is your resistance against gravity. If you need more resistance, use an ankle weight.

REFORMER PILATES

Pilates has a few specific pieces of equipment and classes to target your core

The main piece of equipment in Pilates is called the Reformer. The Reformer is a machine with adjustable springs that allow for progressive resistance. You can find these machines in any Pilates studio, most gyms, and even many rehabilitation clinics. Reformer exercises can seem simple and relaxing because you glide back and forth on the carriage, which makes it a good choice for people with injuries who avoid high-impact exercise. The Reformer has a versatile gliding platform on which you can sit, kneel, stand, or lie on your front, back, or side. To move, you simply push and pull off the foot bar using your arms or legs. Work on the Reformer can be done one-on-one or in a class.

The Reformer

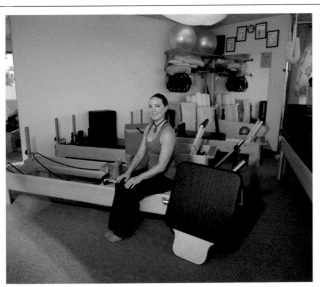

- Pilates classes have become so popular that finding a Reformer near you shouldn't be a challenge.

- Once people love their Pilates exercises, some choose to purchase a Reformer for their home for when they can't get to class or the gym.

- Prices range from between $2,000 to $4,000 for various models of high-quality Reformers. There are home models for less, but they may not be as well built or complete.

- Reformers come in many different colors of upholstery and wood.

Cadillac

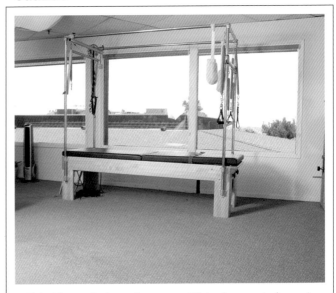

- This 6-foot-tall piece of equipment looks pretty intimidating. Because the Cadillac is such a large piece of equipment, it is rarely used in group classes, so you would need to find a studio that offers private sessions.

- Pilates has created exercises for this machine that can isolate almost every muscle group, so you get a full body workout with a focus on the core.

- This can be a fun and effective way to get results for your midsection.

There is another staple machine in Pilates called the Cadillac. Also known as the Trapeze Table, the Cadillac is used both for exercise and physical therapy. This machine is a raised horizontal tabletop surrounded by a four-poster frame. It features various bars, straps, springs, and levers to create many different kinds of exercises. As with most Pilates equipment, the Cadillac contains various adjustable parts, and you should consult with a trained instructor to teach and guide you through safe, proper usage of each machine as well as proper technique.

Roll Up on Cadillac

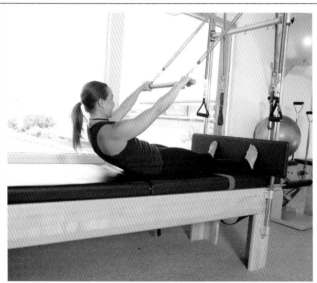

- The roll up is a Pilates exercise that is commonly done as a mat exercise.

- Doing the same exercise on a piece of equipment with different handles and resistance can change what it does and how it feels.

- The bar on the Cadillac will pull you up as you try to roll down. This creates a different resistance than doing it on the mat.

- For balance and variety, do both forms of roll up to warm up the spine and core.

The Benefits of Pilates

- Pilates is a great exercise for anyone with back injuries, because you are lying on your back and have less pressure on your spine.

- Whether mat or Reformer, Pilates will help you focus and control the use of your abs to support your body.

- Pilates was meant to strengthen the spine and core but not to replace basic cardio and resistance training. Adjust your expectations of your goals. Pilates alone may not provide the weight loss you want.

BOXING
A fun workout for the whole torso that promises fast results!

Another way to work the abs while getting amazing cardio and even a little strength training for the upper body is boxing. From jabs, a cross, hooks, and especially an upper cut, boxing utilizes the core to twist, turn, and support your torso as you throw each punch. Every move in boxing requires the abs to work—especially the obliques. Even though the resistance in boxing is not directly on the abs, you use your abs to decelerate your movements.

Learning to use your core to support your body in this movement will be a fun workout for the whole body that can get you results fast! Not too long ago, boxing and kickboxing were a craze. The reason it has quieted down a bit is because people were getting hurt in group fitness, ultrafast class situations. Just like any sport and exercise, there is always a risk of injury when you do not learn and use proper form.

Working one-on-one with a trained professional is best to

The Jab

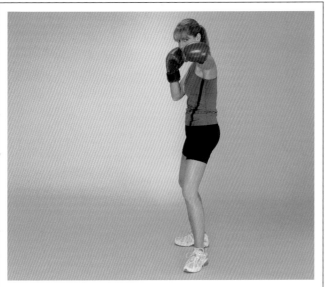

The Cross

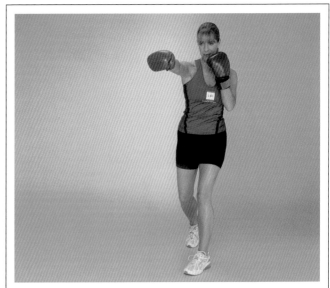

- Start with your hands in front of you, protecting your face.

- Your feet should be at eleven and five o'clock, if you were standing on a clock. The foot that is forward is the arm you will use to jab.

- Use your shoulder, hips, and whole body behind the punch. Stay on the balls of your feet and make sure to keep your knees soft. Never lock out with any joint when throwing a punch.

- The cross is the most powerful punch in boxing—it's the takedown punch.

- In the eleven and five o'clock position, you will punch with the arm opposite the front foot.

- Stay on the ball of your back foot and use your whole body behind this punch.

- Always hit with the front, flat surface of your fist.

perfect your form, but you can get started by learning a few simple hits. Be sure to be prepared before you start, take it slow as you learn good form, and then work up to a greater intensity every few weeks.

The Hook

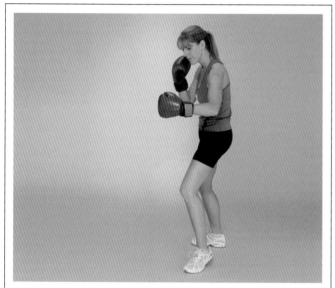

- Use the hook when you are too close to your opponent to extend your arm.

- It's usually a horizontal punch to the rib cage or head with your palm facing you as you throw the punch.

- Like the jab, use one side of your body to provide force behind the punch. Always keep your abs tight to help provide more force.

- Keep you wrist straight—do not flex or bend it when punching.

The Uppercut

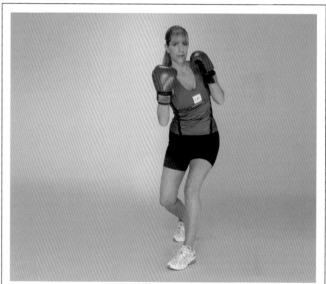

- Like the hook, the uppercut is a punch where you do not fully extend your elbow.

- With this punch, you bend your body to the side and come up from below, because you use this punch when you are too close to fully extend your arms.

- Your palm should face your opponent as you throw an uppercut.

- This can be one of the most powerful punches because the power comes from your legs and torso.

KICKBOXING
Using your core strength with all moves

When designing a new workout program that emphasizes exercises to utilize your abs, thinking outside the box will also help you get creative about ways to use your abs but get a great overall body workout as well. Kickboxing uses the abs to lift the pelvis and legs. You probably will not feel them much in a front kick, but you definitely engage them during a side kick, crescent kick, and roundhouse. Your abs help you lift your pelvis and then leg, so you can produce a strong kick.

Your abs will not automatically work without you thinking about it, however, but learning to use your abs consciously will provide a level of strength you could not achieve without them.

Kickboxing is fun and a great workout that can burn a ton of calories and build leg strength and stamina. As with boxing, this sport requires a skill level to be efficient and effective without injury, so learning correct form is very important.

Front Kick, Mid-Range

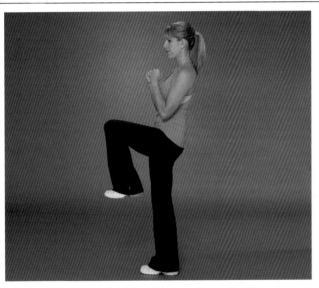

- Start in a lunge position, with one foot in front of the other.

- Keep your arms in a boxing start position to control your torso movement. Both fists should be under your chin with elbows bent.

- Using your back leg, lift your knee up.

- Flex your ankle so when you kick and strike it is with the heel of your foot.

Front Kick, Finish

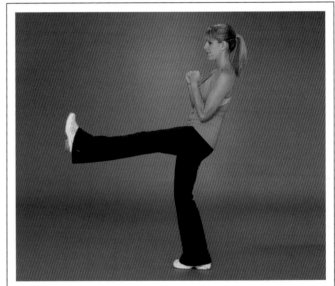

- Keep your abs tight as you pass through each of these positions.

- Imagine the force coming from your butt and hips and passing through your heel to the target.

- When you kick, be sure to push your leg forward as if kicking someone away from you.

- Exhale as you kick, and keep your abs tight; return your leg to the starting position by bending your knee in and then setting it down behind you.

Avoid classes and groups that do all boxing and kickboxing moves too fast. If you feel that you have no control over your moves, you are at greater risk for injury. Once you get the hang of it, you can do it at home with a heavy bag or a standing bag filled with water or sand.

Side Kick, Mid-Range

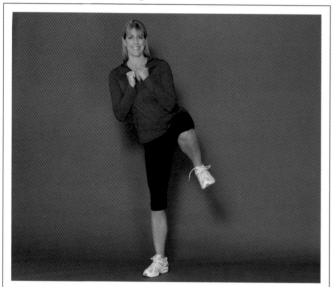

- Start with feet slightly wider than hip width apart.

- Transfer body weight to one side and draw your other leg into the center of your body by bending your knee and hip.

- Keep your feet and knees facing forward and look to the side where you have a target.

- Use your abs to help you balance. Choose a leg and knee height that you can hold and kick from there to start.

Side Kick, Finish

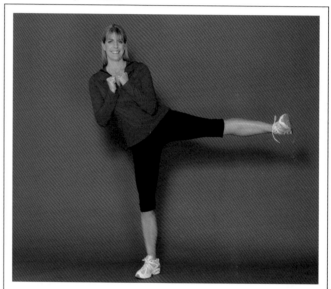

- In a side kick, you kick with the outside of your foot. Strike with the flat part of the side of the foot from the little toes to the heel.

- Concentrate on "pushing" your target away from you when you kick.

- Use your hips and butt to generate your power, not your knee or foot.

- Keep your arms in the center of your body for optimal torso control. And use your abs to create more power.

BODYBLADE

A new oscillating force that uses inertia to create resistance

Because there is no other product like it, I have to introduce you to the Bodyblade, which uses an oscillating force and vibration as the resistance. Body-weight and free-weight exercises use gravity and mass for resistance. Tubing and cables redirect gravity and take out inertia. Bodyblade uses inertia in a balanced way to activate the body in a whole new fashion. Bodyblade is a rapid contraction training tool that has a handle with flexible wings on either side. You create

the amount of resistance by how hard you push or pull—the blade matches you.

Bodyblade is scaled and weighted to flex at 4.5 times per second no matter how hard you drive it. One of the models, a 2.5-pound blade, can generate up to 34 pounds of resistance. This makes Bodyblade a great tool that is versatile and travels well!

You can work all parts of your body with Bodyblade but

Ab Crunch

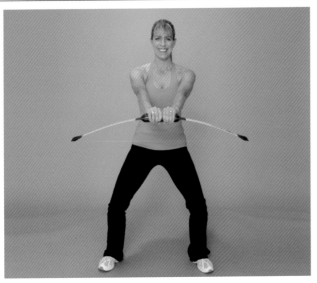

- Place hands side by side in the middle of the blade.

- With your feet wider than shoulder width apart, bend your knees slightly in a small squat.

- Hold the blade so it is parallel to the ground.

- With your palms facing down, push/pull the blade up and down, challenging your core to stay centered.

Ab, Hip, and Thigh Sculptor

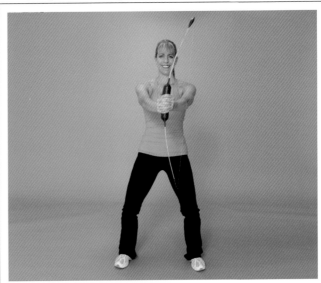

- Grab the Bodyblade with both hands in the middle, with either fingers clasped or hands on top of each other, and hold it vertically.

- With your feet wider than shoulder width apart, bend your knees slightly.

- Extend your arms in front of you with a slight bend.

- Push/pull the blade side to side, challenging your core to stay centered.

will experience a different sensation because the resistance is different. The core gets work at all times because the main thrust of the workout reaches deep to the dynamic stabilizers of the core and builds the body from the center out. This is also a great tool for rehab because it requires no impact.

Intermediate Floor Crunch

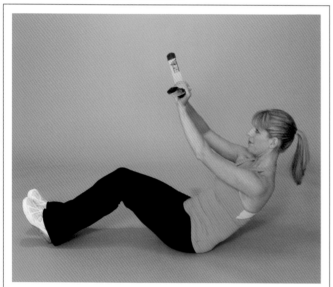

- Assume a mid-range, partial crunch position with your head, chest, and shoulders off the ground and your heels lightly touching the floor for support.

- Hold the Bodyblade in front of your chest in the narrow edge position.

- Rotate the Bodyblade to move up toward the ceiling and down toward the floor for greater support.

- Keep your arms steady, keep breathing, and resist moving!

Lunging Rotational Ab

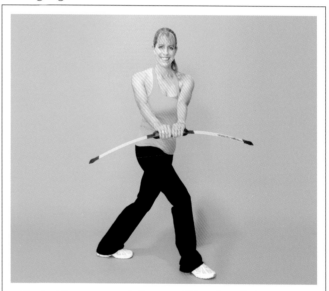

- Start with arms extended out in front of you at shoulder-level height, lunge forward, and rotate to the side of the front foot.

- Keep your palms facing down, while you hold the Bodyblade at chest or navel level.

- This will work the core, hips, inner thighs, and shoulders in both strength and endurance.

- Try moving the blade for 2 to 5 minutes. Start with 2 minutes and work your way up. The more advanced you are, the more time you can sustain.

STABILITY TRAINING

A ball can help increase core strength because you activate your ab muscles to balance

One of the jobs of the abdominal muscles is to hold your pelvis and rib cage together. When you challenge that on an unstable surface, such as a ball or balance board, you add a new kind of force, which can create a great new exercise. In fact, adding the ball to simple daily movements or common exercises will increase your core strength and stability. The ball is a great tool for doing abdominal work, but why not maximize its use by adding the ball and instability to other exercises?

When beginning balance training, I recommend learning how to do each exercise properly and with good form on a solid, stable surface first to gain control. Once you feel you

Sitting

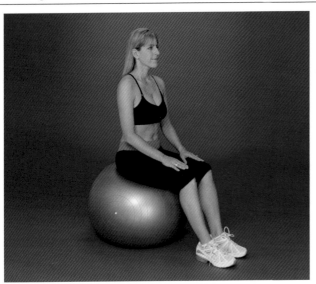

- Know where the center of your ball is. Most have lines that can show you how a ball will roll. Positioning the ball will help it to roll evenly and create a smooth and balanced exercise.

- Sit yourself in the center of the ball with an upright posture.

- Keep your feet flat on the ground and your spine erect.

- Just sitting on the ball for long periods of time will improve your core strength, because you use your abs to keep your balance.

Chest Press

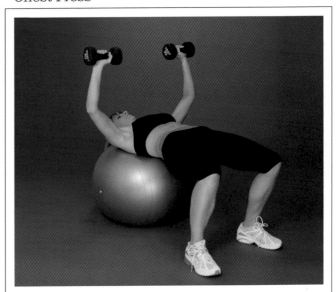

- Lie with your head and shoulders resting on the ball.

- Make sure your hips are in line with your spine and parallel to the floor, with your knees bent and feet flat on the ground.

- Perform a chest press with the same controlled form as you would on a bench or mat. Use lighter weights to start until you become accustomed to the instability.

- Use control because you will have increased range of motion on the ball.

have 100 percent control over the exercise, progress to an unstable surface.

You can add some core strength every day by spending 1 hour sitting on a ball instead of in a chair. This will force you to increase your core's stamina in holding you upright longer. Finding other ways to add small amounts of instability not only engages the abs, but also strengthens your lower body. For example, standing on one foot while brushing your hair or teeth activates your abs, while also strengthening your ankles, hips, and legs.

YELLOW LIGHT

Proceed with small degrees of instability, not large jumps. Give your body time to adapt at each stage and create a solid foundation. One of the easiest ways to get injured is to increase the instability in a difficult exercise before you are ready. Only "load" what you can control. Exercise should be helping you to strengthen your body, not creating injury because of the intensity level.

Bridge

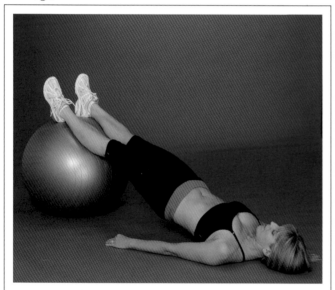

- Lie on your back on the floor.

- Place the ball in front of your legs, find the ball's center, and place a leg on either side of it.

- Make sure your kneecaps and toes face the ceiling. Your legs should be straight on the ball—no bending the knees.

- Concentrate on pulling the back of your knees closer to your butt as you lift your butt in the air.

Shoulder Press

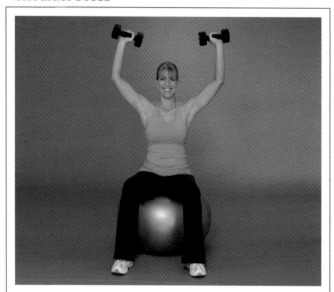

- Sit in the center of the ball.

- Use 3-, 5-, or 8-pound weights to start. In an upright, seated position, lift the weights up and over your head for a shoulder press. Take 2 counts to lift the weights up and 2 counts to bring them back down to your shoulders.

- Your core will work harder to balance your body on the ball as you create force over your head.

- Perform each repetition slowly, concentrating on your core and shoulders.

SWIMMING & POOL TRAINING
A lighter approach for all sizes that is safer on joints

Swimming and pool exercises are great options for the entire body, because the water offers resistance in a way you do not get on land. In gravity we have a direction of resistance—down. With machines, we can change the direction of resistance with pulleys and cams. In water, resistance is consistent in all directions. Most people with injuries or joint problems are told to use a pool for exercise because it is easier on the body due to buoyancy. Without gravity, weight doesn't

matter. Just as with weight training, your muscles contract against resistance, becoming stronger with each session.

There are water exercises to work every muscle group, and the risk of injury is extremely low. Think about exercises you do with free weights. The beauty of resistance training is it can be easily modified. Anything you do with dumbbells can be made into a water exercise. If you already have a routine with free weights, you can create your own water exercises

Treading Water

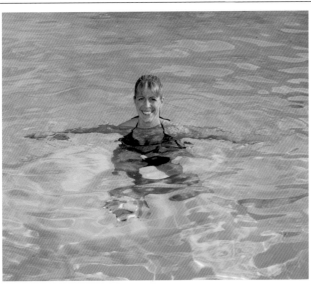

- This is the simplest exercise you can do in the water for your whole body.

- You can tread in any water, but it it's easier in deeper water where your feet do not easily touch the ground.

- Circle your legs around as if you were on a bike. Use your arms to make figure eights right below the surface of the water.

- Your speed is up to you—the faster you go, the more energy you use.

Swimming

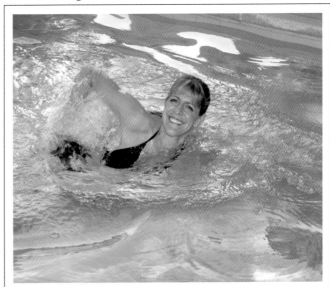

- There are many different strokes you can learn and perform to work all parts of your body.

- The freestyle stroke works the deltoids, hips, quads, and hamstrings, while the butterfly stroke focuses on the complete lower body, deltoids, and chest muscles.

- The breast stroke mainly targets the chest, triceps, and lower body, while also engaging the abs.

- Because the abs have to hold your upper and lower body together while they both move, the core gets a good endurance workout.

that do the same thing. When working out in water, keep your weight distributed evenly and check your posture often. Keep your abs activated and pulled in to support your back. If you have joint issues or just want something different, swimming is great cardio, too.

Water Aerobics

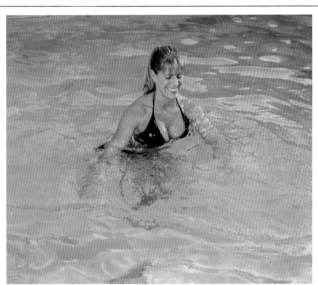

- You can create a water workout using all types of pool equipment—from Styrofoam free weights to buoyancy belts and kickboards.

- Most gyms that have a pool offer water aerobics. Because your balance is challenged in the water,

due to the lack of gravity and added buoyancy, your core works much differently every time you move.

- Most gadgets for the pool come with a DVD or instructions. Check these out if you have a pool at home and want to maximize it.

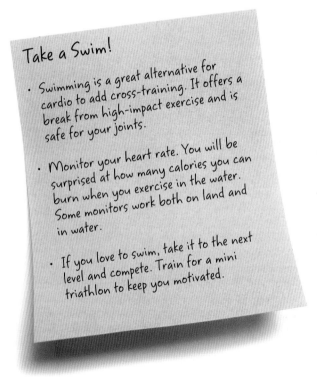

Take a Swim!

- Swimming is a great alternative for cardio to add cross-training. It offers a break from high-impact exercise and is safe for your joints.

- Monitor your heart rate. You will be surprised at how many calories you can burn when you exercise in the water. Some monitors work both on land and in water.

- If you love to swim, take it to the next level and compete. Train for a mini triathlon to keep you motivated.

WORDS TO THE WISE
Why some exercises are dangerous for your spine and joints

Like a building, your body has areas of good and bad weight-baring options. We often do exercises without considering if the force we are applying to our body is to a joint that can handle it. When it comes to the abs, we have to consider the spine. In today's world, where many people complain of back problems, it is wise to choose exercises that offer maximum benefit with the least amount of risk. All joints are susceptible to injury by exercise if precautions are not taken.

On these pages we will review common exercises that put the spine at high risk. Most people do not consider their joints when building an exercise program or choosing proper form, because they cannot see their joints. That is why I named my company Invisible Fitness, because we care about creating programs that not only get you results but also protect your joints, not deteriorate them faster.

Some common high-risk exercises are deadlifts, triceps

The Spine

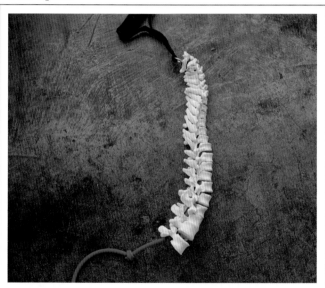

- There are thirty-three vertebrae in your spine from neck to pelvis.

- Every two vertebrae make a joint, so throughout the entire spine you have many joints, which can move independently.

- The bones toward the neck, called the cervical vertebrae, are smaller and have more motion, making them less stable. The vertebrae get thicker and larger as you move down the spine, making the lumbar vertebrae more stable and less mobile. Use caution to not force extra movement in the lower spine.

The Shoulder Joint

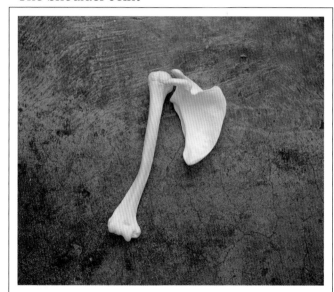

- The shoulder joint consists of the humerus and scapula.

- Notice that the head of the humerus is larger than the socket it is attached to—this makes it very mobile and not so stable.

- Your soft tissue and muscle are what create the integrity of this joint, because there is no bone holding it together.

- Shoulder injuries are very common because people often place too much load or force on this unstable joint.

dips, walking lunges, and upright rows. There are many movements people make in the gym to mirror movements in life, like a golf swing with a free weight. I would consider that dangerous and not a good choice for cross-training for golf, because the forces are distributed differently.

GREEN ● LIGHT

If you want to strengthen your shoulder to last longer and be stronger in golf, work all the other muscles around the joint that support it and do not get used in the actual sport. This will help to stabilize and protect your shoulder because you create balanced strength.

BE CAREFUL!

The Knee Joint

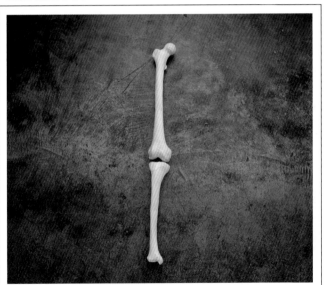

- The knee is a hinge joint like the hinge of a door—it moves in two directions only.

- Because the knee connects the upper leg to the lower leg, it absorbs all the force from the hips and pelvis as well as the feet and ankles.

- The knee only flexes and extends; it should not rotate. Injury often occurs in the knee with a sudden change of direction or twisting of the knee.

- The knees can be easily susceptible to injury and wear and tear.

Protecting Your Joints

- Everyone has a different structure, so there is no one-size-fits-all solution.

- If you are not sure about an exercise, always do it very slowly, with control.

- Make sure to think about the muscles you are contracting and imagine it pulling you—not throwing you.

- Pay attention to your body and how it feels. Recognize the difference between muscle fatigue and joint pain.

NO NEED FOR BROOMSTICKS

If your resistance uses gravity, swinging side to side is a waste of time

I often see people in the gym put a bar on their back and start swinging side to side. Let us review the basics of physics, gravity, and anatomy. If I am standing upright without a machine, I am most likely going to do a gravity-based exercise, because gravity pulls down. If I place a broomstick or bar on my shoulders, that will only add more weight that pulls

down. If I want to work my obliques, I may think that rotating side to side will work them, but the resistance I am using does not match the motion I am making. In order to effectively add resistance to a muscle, it has to be in the same plane of motion in the opposite direction. The plane of motion in this case is horizontal—I am moving side to side. The direction of

Broomstick Swing = Bad Idea

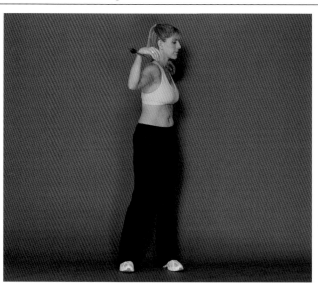

- This is a common position I see people take when they want to work their obliques.

- If you want to add resistance to twisting, use a cable or tubing positioned to pull you in the opposite direction you are twisting.

- Twisting in general is a dangerous exercise, because most people use speed instead of control.

- Allow your abs to work naturally in twisting motions like those used in boxing or swimming; save broomsticks for cleaning.

Punch and Twist

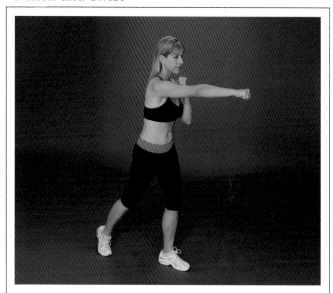

- Many aerobic and boxing classes use punching from side to side to warm up.

- This can be a safe exercise to do because the lower body follows the upper body naturally.

- When you lock the bottom half and move the top half, you risk injury if you do too much.

- Remember that you can't spot reduce, so aim to do all kinds of motions for a balanced workout.

my resistance is vertical, however, with gravity pulling down so my resistance is not being applied to my motion, making the bar or broomstick useless. This can also be dangerous depending on how much extra weight is on your shoulders.

Now, we also need to talk about control, momentum, and deceleration. For optimal control over your muscles, you want to contract them by "pulling." Your muscle will never pull you into a dangerous place, but you can be thrown into one. Using the force generated by twisting with a weight on your shoulders creates a momentum that your muscles

and joints have to stop—this can put wear and tear on your joints. In this example, the joints in question are the joints of your spine. If the weight is heavy enough, there will be more force generated by your body to stop your spine from twisting past what it can handle than by actually working the muscles to make them stronger. The bottom line? Stay away from exercises that may look like this.

Lateral Bend

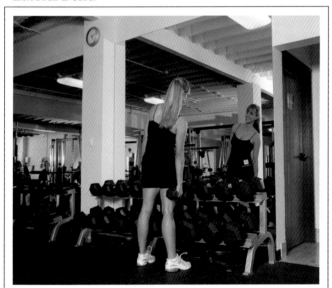

- Recalling that spot reducing does not exist, use this exercise with light weights when you want to stimulate some new fibers in your abs.

- Hold a light to medium weight for you in your hand and allow your arm to take your rib cage to a side bend

on the side that is holding the weight.

- Concentrate on pulling yourself up with the opposite side. Your opposite ribs will pull you back in to neutral.

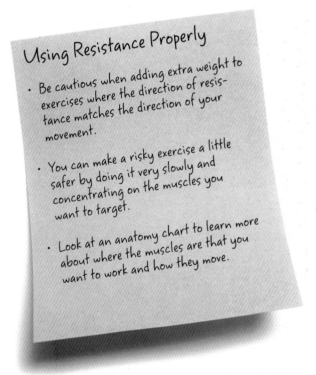

Using Resistance Properly

- Be cautious when adding extra weight to exercises where the direction of resistance matches the direction of your movement.

- You can make a risky exercise a little safer by doing it very slowly and concentrating on the muscles you want to target.

- Look at an anatomy chart to learn more about where the muscles are that you want to work and how they move.

LEG THROW = DANGEROUS

Someone else throwing your legs may be too much too soon with serious risk to the spine

When I see a trainer or workout partner throwing the legs of someone on the floor, I want to cringe. And the sad part is that I used to love this exercise—until I learned anatomy and force. This is a hard exercise, and that is why people like it—they feel it. But do they feel it in the right place?

This common exercise relies on the partner or trainer to use his or her force to throw a person's legs toward the floor. The first problem is that we cannot measure the amount of force used by the person throwing the legs. This becomes an issue because he or she most likely will not be able to repeat the same force over and over again. With exercise, you want to make sure to control your forces so you know when you

Leg Throw, Start

- This exercise typically starts with you grabbing your trainer's ankles while he or she grabs yours.

- You can do this exercise in such a way as to apply very little force so that it is safer.

- By keeping your back flat on the ground while decelerating your legs, you keep the force out of your spine and direct it to the ab muscles.

- If you're not an advanced exerciser, I would not even put your lower back at risk with this exercise.

Leg Throw, Finish

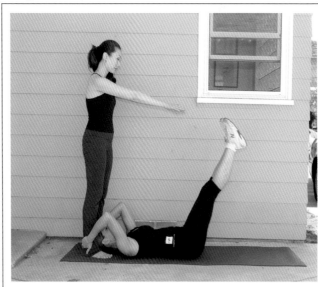

- You do not know or cannot control how much force is being used on you.

- To compensate for too much force, the spine lifts up and helps decelerate the legs, putting pressure on your lower back.

- Because this is usually a difficult exercise, people often "feel" it, so they think it's a good exercise.

- If you can keep your back on the ground, you protect your back and actually use your abs.

improve. If the force is different each time, you may not know if you are improving.

The second problem with this exercise is that you do not know how much force the person doing the exercise can take. When you use reps, sets, and even weights in exercise, you can test the level that is appropriate for your strength level. When you do this exercise, you may work too much too soon and not know it until you are injured.

The third problem with this exercise is that most people do it so their abs decelerate the force provided by the partner or trainer, and often they absorb this force in their backs and spines. Without having control over the force, when the lower back lifts off the ground, the person doing the exercise is actually absorbing the forces in the spine, not the abs. This can cause an injury very quickly or exacerbate an existing condition.

Assisted Isometric Start

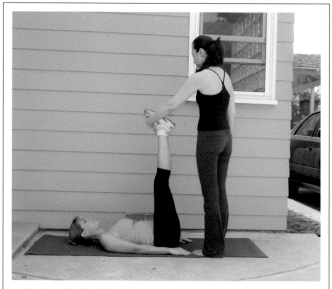

- Replace the leg throw with an isometric version.

- Hold your legs in the same position and keep your lower back on the ground.

- Think of pulling your pelvis in to your ribs as in a lower crunch.

- Make sure to breathe in and out as you do this exercise; do not hold your breath.

Assisted Isometric End

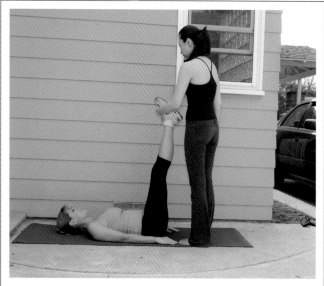

- Hold your legs in the same position; keep your lower back on the ground.

- Have your trainer or partner pull you slightly away from your center using minimal force.

- Have him or her maintain the same amount pressure, if possible, as you resist his or her pulling your legs away from you.

- Adjust the level so you feel a difficulty of a 6 to 8 on a scale of 10. Hold it for 45 to 90 seconds and do 2 to 3 sets.

CHAIRS ARE FOR SITTING

How to use a Roman chair properly so you don't damage your spine

A piece of exercise equipment known as the Roman chair was developed for advanced exercisers to work their backs, not their abs. However, I see many people doing all kinds of crunches on this piece. This can be very dangerous for two reasons. First, you have an enormous range of motion. Because your legs are locked and your spine held in a diagonal position with no boundaries, you can move a great deal in any direction. Having more motion is not always a good

thing, however. The weight of your body becomes the resistance, so how much you weigh from the waist up will determine how heavy the load is.

The second reason this exercise can be dangerous is inertia. Because you are in a diagonal position to start, gravity wants to pull you down at all times. You have to have a strong back and spinal muscles just to hold yourself up, as well as strong hamstrings to keep your legs in place.

Roman Chair Back Exercise

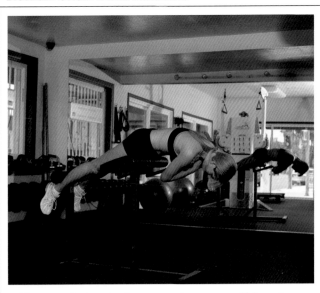

- Place your feet under the pads to secure your body on the machine.

- Start with a straight back and activate your glutes and hips to keep you stabilized.

- Release your back, one vertabra at a time, and

lower yourself down in a bend, spinal flexed position keeping your pelvis stabilized.

- Once you are bent over in a range that is comfortable, start to come back up again—one vertebra at a time—until your back is straight.

Roman Chair Hamstring Exercise

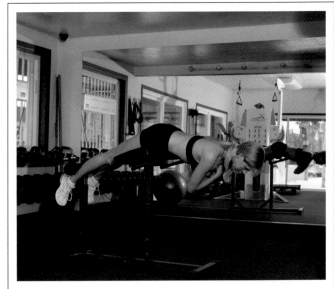

- You can use the Roman chair to work your hamstrings, too.

- Follow the beginning directions to the left, but instead of bending your spine, keep it straight.

- Using your abs and spinal muscles to keep yourself straight, release your glutes and allow your hips to flex forward.

- Allow your body to bend at the hips only as far as you can handle and then visualize your hamstrings pulling you back up into place.

Choosing an exercise like this requires a solid foundation of strength and stamina. Know when you are choosing a high-risk exercise that you may not get any greater benefit than if you did a lower risk exercise.

················· RED ● LIGHT ·················

If you have back or hip problems, do not attempt this exercise. I would advise that you not do side bends or twisting on this machine in order to work your abs. Do only what you can control, keep the range of motion small and controlled to start, and increase it as you gain strength and stamina.

BE CAREFUL!

Abs Sling

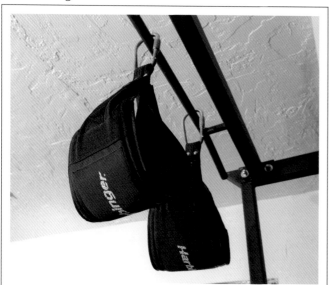

- Another highly advanced exercise is doing lower crunches with a sling.

- Your arms go through the sling, which helps to hold up your body weight so you can do a reverse crunch in the air.

- What the abs are mostly doing is supporting you with an isometric contraction.

- Be sure not to use momentum and jump into a lower crunch; really work on pulling yourself there properly.

Protect Your Spine

- You can find many tools to help create different ab exercises.

- Some of them rely on momentum and speed and can be dangerous for your spine.

- Whatever you try, make sure you are at a fitness level that is ready for higher risk exercises.

- Remember that when you contract your abs they pull you into spinal flexion. Make sure your resistance matches your motion.

YOUR LEGS AS WEIGHTS

You can use your legs as resistance as long as you prepare for each stage of difficulty

For a lot of ab exercises on the floor and in other positions, your legs act as the weight or resistance. I do body-weight exercises with both my male and female clients, because most people do not practice using their own body to provide resistance. Using your body as your resistance is great for creating workouts you can do at home, outside, or when you travel with little or no equipment needed.

Lower body and ab exercises are easy to create because the legs offer a variety of levels of resistance. Leg positions on the ground can vary based on the movements you want to make, but one thing remains the same: The position of your legs will affect the difficulty of the exercise. Because we work

KNACK ABSOLUTE ABS

Legs in Neutral

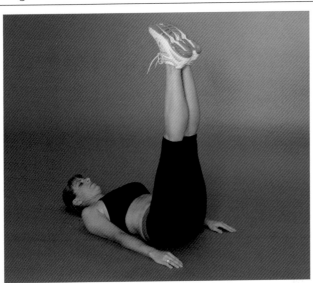

- When it comes to the resistance on your abs and back, having your legs straight up is considered neutral.

- In this position your quads and hip flexors work hard to hold up your legs.

- Your hamstrings are being asked to relax and stretch to allow your legs to be in this position.

- Because your legs are in line with gravity, they offer very little resistance to your abs or back in this position.

Legs at 45 Degrees

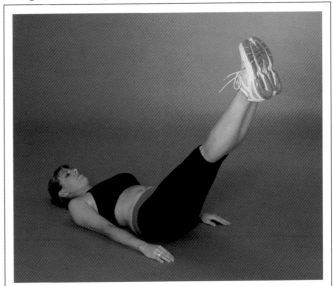

- The more perpendicular you are to gravity, the greater the resistance.

- You should only use this position if you can keep your lower back on the ground.

- The length of your legs and torso determine how difficult each place in the range of motion is for you.

- Use your abs to keep your pelvis and rib cage together. If your lower back comes off the ground, the resistance is too much for you.

with gravity, the angle of your body and the position in which you hold your legs determine how much resistance you create with the weight of your legs. There are ways to make body-weight exercises easier or harder, but I want you to understand how holding your legs while lying on the ground affects you. I create beginner, intermediate, and advanced versions of the same exercise by changing the leg position.

Tabletop

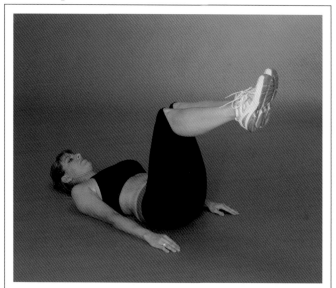

- Bending the legs cuts the resistance in half, because you have shortened the lever.

- For optimal resistance keep your ankles above your knees to decrease force to your back.

- You can move your legs closer to you or farther away to change the level of resistance. The farther away you go, the harder it will be.

- Maintain contact between your lower back and the floor to control and use your abs to hold you together.

When Legs Are Too Much

- You can tell when the weight of your legs is too much for you when you lift your back off the ground.

- The force is absorbed and now stopped by your spine instead of your muscles.

- You may also start to feel a strain or pull in your back before it lifts off the ground, in which case you want to bring your legs closer to you.

- Be sure to do these movements slowly with control.

79

USING SPEED
Speed is not your friend . . . yet

You should plan when to use speed during exercise. When you do an exercise quickly, you should utilize muscle fibers that are already good at that particular motion. If you try to do an exercise too quickly, however, you may not be able to "listen" to your body, because the speed may mask any warning signals it sends you. This communication with your body is called biofeedback. Biofeedback is any signal from your body that tells you when things are too intense. Pain is a

form of biofeedback. Generally, when you do things quickly, you lose good form. I see many people doing resistance exercises with speed to "get it done," so I want to explain an important concept in resistance training. Failure is the goal in building muscle. This is when you work slowly on the muscle and for enough time to fatigue it to a level we call failure. There are physiological profiles for all kinds of desired goals, like building muscle, explosive strength, and endurance.

How to Train for Speed

- When training for speed, start slowly and work your way up.

- Use resistance that is not gravity based to protect your joints while training. Tubing, cables, and water are great choices.

- Make sure to train all the muscles around the joint that you wish to move faster.

- Cross-train for muscular balance and always be mindful and body aware. Your body will tell you when it does not like something you are doing.

Muscle Sprain

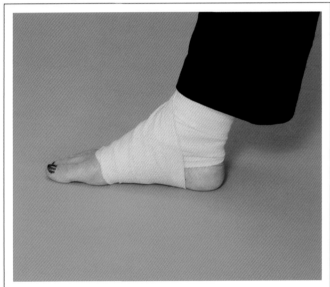

- Speed often does not focus on control of muscles, but instead on control and focus of movement, so if your muscles are not 100 percent prepared, you could cause a muscle sprain.

- A muscle sprain is a tear in the soft tissue that results

when the force applied to it was too much for it to handle.

- Often, the only way to heal a sprain is with time.

- To reduce inflammation and speed up healing , I recommend acupuncture and taking extra fish oil.

When it comes to deciding how fast or slow to perform an exercise, knowing or consulting with someone can help you determine the most effective way to do an exercise. When it comes to ab work, slower is usually better, but be careful not to rest too much in between reps.

Using numbers to guide how many repetitions you do for a set of exercises is a good way to get started but sometimes leads to people doing them too fast to get them over with. Try slowing down your exercises to a 4- to 6-second rep speed with no resting during the set. Try doing constant, slow motion in your exercise for 45 to 90 seconds. Test out which intensity level is right for you to get started.

Neck Pain

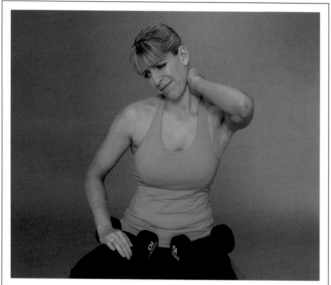

- Using speed to work your abs can result in a pulled or strained neck. This is the most common complaint with a bad ab routine.

- When you concentrate on going fast, you sometimes forget to use good form.

- The head and neck get pulled on first when you lose good form, due to fatigue or lack of concentration on your form.

- If doing abs quickly is a goal, work up to it by starting slowly and always using proper form.

Back Pain

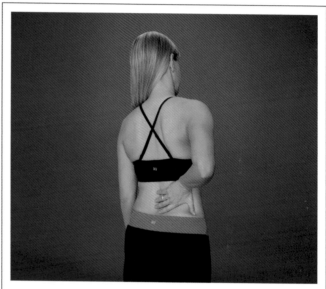

- Back pain is so common these days that we cannot chance getting injured in our workouts.

- Because the lower back stretches when you contract your abs in spinal flexion, you may feel something in the lower back.

- If you sit all day and always have a tight lower back, your back may not want to lengthen when you do abs, and this could cause discomfort.

- Using speed will not help alleviate back pain but could help create more discomfort.

AVOIDING SHOULDER INJURIES
Boxing with weights is a huge no-no for any goal

When exercises become too easy, most people want to add weights to the motion. As discussed earlier with the broomstick, you need to know whether or not the resistance you have added is actually being applied to the exercise you are doing. Boxing is a cardio sport with short bursts of energy and power. The average boxing round is 3 minutes. Boxing can also offer resistance benefits to back muscles, shoulders, arms, and abs. As your body adapts to boxing, it gets easier

and you get stronger and faster.

If you box to build your arms, you are doing the wrong exercise. Adding free weights to a boxing routine is the fastest way to ruin your shoulders. Remember: The weight pulls down thanks to gravity. When you punch, you create a horizontal motion forward and back, not up and down. So the weight in your hands is only challenging your shoulder's ability to hold itself in place. And remember what the shoulder

Shoulder Joint in Flexion

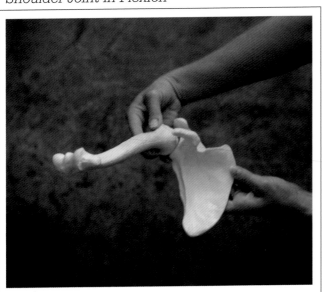

- The humerus—the arm bone—is very easily moved out and around the shoulder girdle.

- To keep the shoulder strong, it is important to strengthen the muscles that stabilize and move it. Your chest, back, trapezius, deltoids, triceps, biceps, and

rotator cuff muscles all help to stabilize the shoulder.

- Because of the way it is built, it is very easy to injure the shoulder.

- Physical therapists have cited shoulder impingement as one of the five most common injuries they see.

Boxing with Tubing—Jab

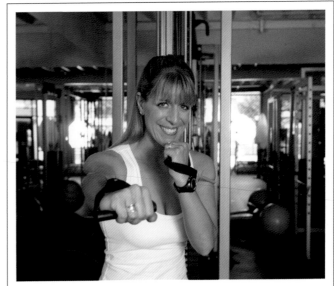

- If you want to increase the speed or strength of a punch, you can add resistance with tubing or elastic bands.

- You need to anchor the tubing onto a doorstop, post, or tree at shoulder level to perform this exercise.

- Match the height of the tubing to your range of motion so you can effectively resist the motions you're going to make.

- Since gravity is not involved here, you can use speed to find new ways to train this motion.

joint looks like? It is very mobile, not very stable, and is only held together by soft tissue and muscle. When you accelerate the weight forward and do not release it, your ligaments and muscles have to decelerate your arm to keep it from flying off your body. You will most likely experience joint degeneration as well as muscle tears and ligament strains. Why chance the wear and tear on the shoulder when you can choose a different exercise that can better build the muscle more safely?

And for every sport, adding weight to the same motions you make while playing that sport is usually not the best way to train. Find exercises that compliment the sport and match your movements with resistance in the same plane of motion.

Boxing with Tubing—Cross

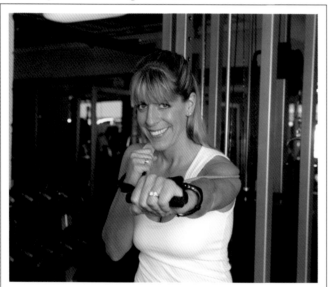

- You can add resistance to all boxing motions with tubing.

- You may need to change the height of the tubing to match your punch, whether it be a jab/cross or a hook or uppercut.

- You can start off with lighter tubing to get used to the resistance; increase the thickness as you get stronger.

- When working with both sides of the body, you might need to secure to points on both sides of you to provide resistance appropriately.

Adding Resistance Safely

- Be careful when you add weights to any exercise.

- If gravity is your main direction, try different kinds of resistance with which to cross-train.

- Tubing and cables and swimming and vibration can enhance a workout and increase your fitness level more safely then adding more free weights.

- Pay attention to how your body responds to an exercise as you do it and then 24 to 48 hours later. Pain and pinching may indicate a problem.

CARDIO BASICS

It's all about endurance—try jumping rope or jumping jacks for a change of pace

Cardiovascular exercise is often defined as a low level of resistance exercise that you can do for an extended duration. More simply put, it's easy enough for your muscles to do for a long time. Common forms of cardio include walking, running, hiking, biking, boxing, dancing, swimming, jumping rope, performing jumping jacks, doing aerobic tapes and classes, indoor group cycling, playing tennis, and so on.

What defines effective or efficient cardio is based on the intensity level. If you start a walking program for a few weeks after being sedentary, you will most likely see some results. After your body has adjusted to this exercise, you will plateau. When the body gets better at executing an exercise program,

Jump Rope, Start

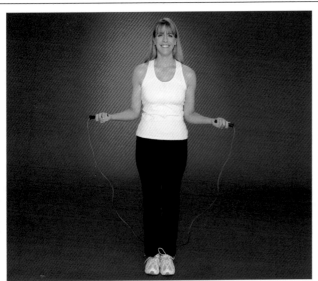

Jump Rope, Finish

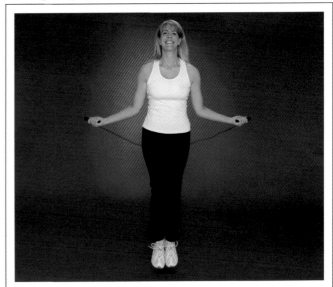

- Use a rope that's not too long or too short. You can find ropes in the gym or invest in one that travels with you.

- When the handles are in your hands and your elbows are bent, the rope should just touch the ground. If the rope is too long, it will drag on the floor and be harder to use.

- Start with your feet together and knees slightly bent.

- Squeeze your abs while doing the exercise and remember to breathe.

- Keep your feet and legs together when you jump. You can do a single bounce or a double bounce where you jump twice before the rope circles around you.

- Soften your knees on the way down; do not land with locked knees.

- Make small circles with the rope to start and keep your elbows by your sides.

- Start with 1 to 5 minutes and gradually increase your time by 1-minute increments. Set a goal to reach 15 minutes.

it's called adaptation. As you adapt, the exercises get easier, therefore the body does not need to change.

The best way to monitor your cardio to make sure it is challenging enough for your body to lose weight, get stronger, and build endurance is to track your heart rate either manually or with a monitor. I call cardio exercise your "short-term investment strategy." Cardiovascular exercise generally does not build muscle, does not build bone, and does not increase your metabolism. You burn calories when you do it—and maybe for a short time after—and that is it. In order for it to keep working, you have to keep doing it. Cardio burns calories in the moment, increases stamina, and can lower blood pressure and improve heart and lung capacity.

Cardio exercise is important, but how often, how much, and what type to do depend on you and your goals. I will give you a formula for figuring that out later in the book. You can do cardio anywhere—at home, the gym, or even when traveling. All you need is your heart rate monitor and some good shoes and supportive clothes.

Jumping Jack, Start

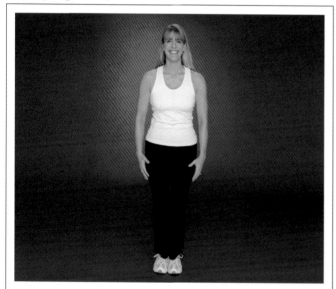

- Start with your feet flat on the ground and knees slightly bent.

- Remember to squeeze your abs throughout the entire exercise.

- Start in an upright posture, chest up and shoulders back.

- For some women, using the arms in a full range of motion over the head can make certain parts jiggle too much. You can choose to do half of the range by lifting your arms just to shoulder height.

Jumping Jack, Finish

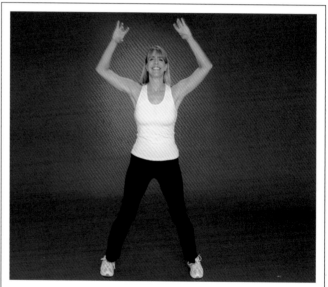

- Jump with your feet slightly wider than hip width apart and land toward the balls of your feet. Keep your knees soft—do not lock them.

- You can do a set of jumping jacks anywhere, so do a few sets throughout the day to get started.

- Start slowly and do not rush. Precision with placing your feet and using your abs is important.

- Start with 30 to 50 reps and increase gradually. Record your progress so you can see yourself improve.

HEART RATE TRAINING

Knowing your heart rate not only keeps you safe, it also helps you track your progress

Most of us determine an exercise's difficulty by our own perception. And there is even a scale to measure that, called RPE—rate of perceived exertion. We use a scale of 1 to 10, with 10 as the difficulty near failure. The problem with our perception is that it is skewed. Depending on body awareness, some people have no idea how to read what is

happening inside their bodies. Some people believe if they sweat, they must be working hard. What happens when you are outside in the heat and sweat? This is not a good way to gauge your exercise intensity.

If you have any heart problems, have a lot of stress, or know that you have little body awareness, using a heart rate

Heart Rate Monitor

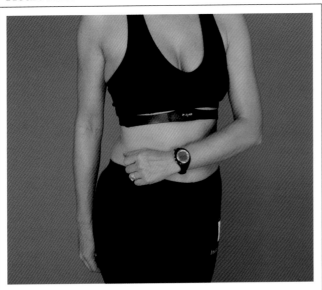

- Most heart rate monitors are made up of two pieces: the watch and the chest strap.

- The chest strap should fit under your sports bra or rib cage; keep it tight enough to keep it from moving.

- The watch reads the heart rate from the chest strap and gives you constant feedback about where you are in terms of intensity level.

- I recommend using both pieces when you do cardio to track your progress.

The Watch

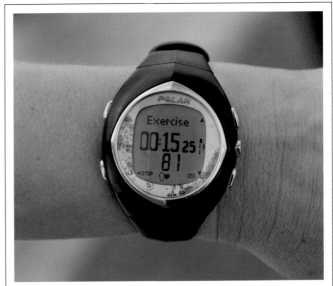

- There are many models and brands of heart rate monitors.

- Depending on the model, the watch will give you information on heart rate, calories burned, and maximum and average heart rate.

- You can use a heart rate monitor at the gym, at home, or outside, and it can give you a summary of your workout.

- The watch displays your heart rate, which can also help you determine when you are doing too much.

monitor can help you be safe with exercise. If you are a seasoned exerciser, this tool is important to help you get past a plateau and track your efficiency on a regular basis. Most of the women I have coached and trained over the years who were frustrated about exercise had not tracked when their bodies became strong enough for their chosen exercise. People waste a lot of time not knowing whether or not their exercise is working.

Using a heart rate monitor is also a safety tool. One time I was working out when I noticed my heart rate was higher than I thought it should be, and I found out I had a fever. Had I not known by the feedback on the monitor that something was off, I might have pushed myself harder and become injured. This tool can only help you and give you great information. For maximum safety and efficiency in your workout, do not underestimate how a tracking device can help you.

Taking Your Pulse

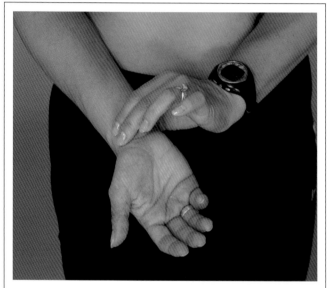

- You can manually check your heart rate before, during, and after exercise.

- Using your first and second fingers, press firmly on the indentation just below the thumb on the wrist.

- Start counting with 0 on the first beat and watch the clock for 6 seconds.

- Add a 0 to that number. This is your approximate heart rate.

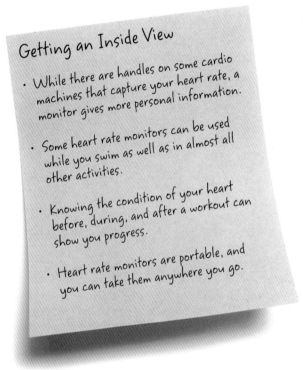

Getting an Inside View

- While there are handles on some cardio machines that capture your heart rate, a monitor gives more personal information.

- Some heart rate monitors can be used while you swim as well as in almost all other activities.

- Knowing the condition of your heart before, during, and after a workout can show you progress.

- Heart rate monitors are portable, and you can take them anywhere you go.

INTERVAL TRAINING

Advanced levels can see faster fat burning because of the increase in intensity

There are two major types of cardio training: steady state and interval training. These days most fitness professionals—and wellness medical professionals too—quote research that says high-intensity interval training is more effective at burning fat. Is this true? It can be for some people. But what is true for everyone is that what you do often, and then adapt to,

will eventually stop working and not help you to the same results as it once did. This applies to every kind of exercise.

If you have done cardio exercise in a steady state—that is, you have maintained the same or similar intensity level for the duration of a workout—it may be time to try some interval training. I must caution you, however, that you first want

Running and Sprints

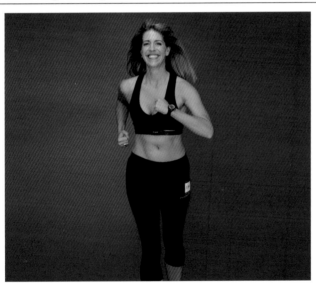

- The most convenient exercise for interval training is running or sprints.

- Make sure when you start that you have no pain or injuries that could become aggravated by increasing your speed.

- In a 30-minute example, run or sprint as hard as you can comfortably (no joint pain) for 1 to 2 minutes.

- Follow that sprint by walking or slowing your pace for 5 to 8 minutes, then repeat. Gradually increase your sprint or run time by 1 to 2 minutes.

Cycling

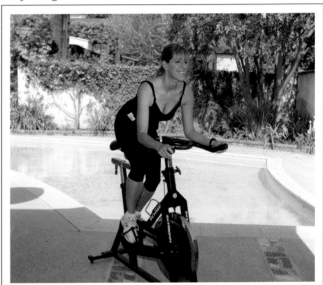

- Indoor group cycling classes offer interval training in a class setting.

- Jumping, running, and sprints are usually added throughout a class, which change your level of intensity.

- I have a spin bike and create my own intervals when I exercise on it.

- Remember to alternate between high-intensity work for up to 3 minutes with periods of lower intensity work that you can sustain for 5 to 15 minutes or more.

to prepare your body for higher levels of work. If you are a beginner exerciser, I might not recommend sprints. You may want to train with steady-state running or jogging and gradually increase your speed before using high bursts of speed in a sprint. If you are an intermediate or advanced exerciser who has strength and some balance as a good foundation, it may be time to add high-intensity bursts into your routine.

You can turn any cardio that you are currently doing into an interval-training exercise by using high-intensity, short-term bursts of activity. If you walk or jog on the treadmill for 20 or 30 minutes, for example, and you're not seeing great results, try sprinting for 1 to 2 minutes every 5 to 8 minutes. The goal is to increase your heart rate quickly and sustain it for 1 to 2 minutes until you cannot do it any longer. Then you take 5 to 10 minutes to recover and repeat. Spin classes have built-in intervals just like boxing.

Elliptical Trainer

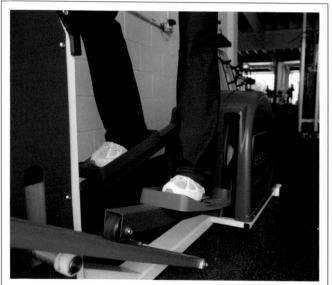

- The elliptical trainer is often suggested for people with knee problems because it offers a low-impact workout.

- You can create intervals on an elliptical just as you can on a spin bike.

- Time yourself for 1 minute and focus on moving your legs fast without bouncing.

- Alternate between 1- or 2-minute blasts of intensity with no bounce and the easy running-like motion you can make on the elliptical to create a new kind of cardio for you.

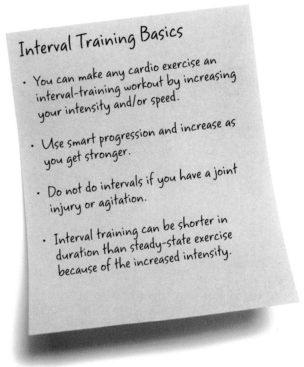

Interval Training Basics

- You can make any cardio exercise an interval-training workout by increasing your intensity and/or speed.

- Use smart progression and increase as you get stronger.

- Do not do intervals if you have a joint injury or agitation.

- Interval training can be shorter in duration than steady-state exercise because of the increased intensity.

BOOSTING METABOLISM
Use resistance training to build muscle and boost metabolism

Metabolism is based on two major components: your nervous system and your muscles. Your nervous system needs energy all day long, and whether you have a "type A" or a "surfer dude" personality will determine how much energy you need each day. On these pages, we will concentrate on the muscular system.

Muscle is active tissue; fat is not. The more muscle you have, the more energy you need. Building muscle—and I do not mean bodybuilder style—increases your metabolism, builds bone, and is your long-term investment strategy. When you have a higher metabolism, it is easier for you to maintain and lose weight.

Within your genetic structure, you have muscles that you do not use on a regular basis. Activating those muscles and increasing their abilities can help turn flabby parts into firm parts.

Legs

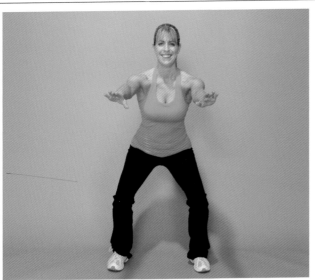

- Working your legs with resistance training is the fastest way to reduce body fat and increase metabolism.

- Because your legs support you every day, working the legs can burn a great deal of calories and also provide a little cardio.

- Many people mistake cardio for leg training. Cardio work does not build muscle.

- Building muscle in your legs will make cardio easier and increase your ability to do higher intensity exercises (which can burn more calories!).

Upper Body

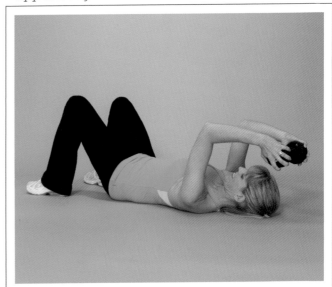

- Building muscle and strength in the upper body is important not only for a balanced-looking physique but for injury prevention as you age.

- Muscles move bone and stabilize the body, so when you age and lose strength, common movements become harder to do.

- A balanced program works your back, chest, shoulders, and arms.

- Building muscle in your whole body increases your metabolism and helps you burn more calories every day.

For long-term results resistance training must be part of your exercise program. Recall that in resistance training, you add resistance to a motion so that it becomes intense enough to create fatigue and failure. If the exercise is not difficult enough, there is no reason for the body to change. Many women I have worked with do not fully understand their threshold for resistance training.

Core Training

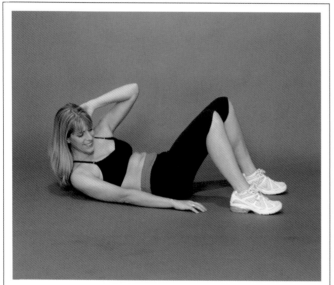

- Because the abs act as stabilizers for the body—holding the upper and lower body together—your focus should not be on building them the same way you build the upper or lower body.

- Work your abs every time you perform an upper and lower body exercise. Remember to activate them!

- Working just your abs will not increase your metabolism.

Balance Training

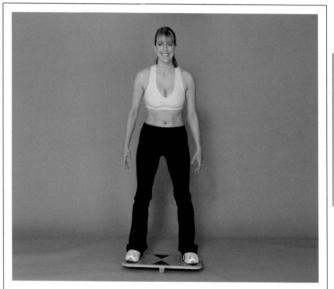

- Every resistance-training program should include some balance training.

- Working on your balance increases the strength and stability of all the small muscle groups that support the joints.

- As we age, we lose the ability to balance well if we do not practice.

- Balance training helps create a solid foundation for more intense workouts.

OTHER FACTORS

What else contributes to building muscle and burning calories?

If losing weight and maintaining good health were as simple as math, we would all be perfect, right? Unfortunately they're not that easy. In addition to exercise and nutrition, there are other factors involved that can help—or hurt—your chances of reaching your goals. Hormones, genetics, the nervous system, and lifestyle factors all play a role in weight loss and overall health. There are so many factors in health and weight loss that create results, that people are often overwhelmed and discouraged when unrealistic expectations are not met.

How old are you? Have you been a constant exerciser? Do you work a sedentary job? Look at your family tree to understand your genetics. How does that affect you? Establish your goals based on all the factors in your life and develop a program that you can take step by step with realistic expectations. Counting calories—both in what you eat and how much you burn—gives you only a partial picture of the

Hormones

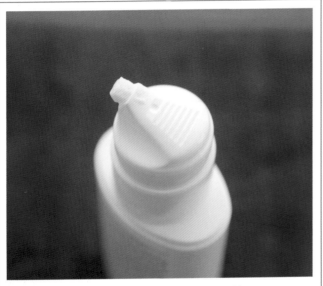

- Testosterone is a hormone that helps build and maintain muscle mass. Men generally have more testosterone than women.

- As you age, if you do not replace your hormones, they decrease along with your ability to hold onto muscle tissue.

- Bioidentical hormone replacement therapy can help balance your body chemistry as well as build and maintain a higher metabolism. Check with an anti-aging doctor for more information.

Genetics

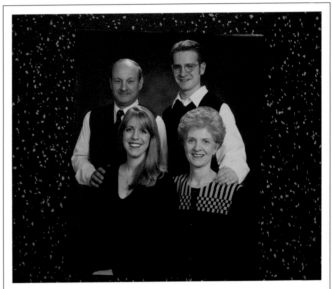

- Some people are born with a faster nervous system and metabolism than others.

- Body types and how you build muscle are also genetic and can affect how well you burn calories.

- Our skeletal structures are all built differently; this can dictate what kinds of exercises best suit us.

- Like it or not, your genetics play a big role in how your body responds to exercise.

factors that contribute to your weight loss or lack there of. If you are having a hard time losing weight, and you know how many calories you take in, look at the other factors listed here.

ZOOM

Your resting metabolism is how many calories you burn at rest and is based on how much active tissue you have. Get your body fat checked and factor that in, too. You may think you burn more than you actually do. That is the most common reason women, especially, have difficulty losing weight Consult a trainer or nutritionist to figure out your resting metabolism.

The Nervous System

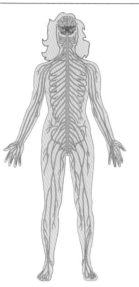

- The nervous system needs energy to control the body and brain.

- Whether it is astrological or genetic, some people naturally have more energy than others.

- A faster nervous system may burn more calories, but it can also create more stress. Some people with lots of energy can also burn out more easily.

- Having a slower nervous system can be a gift, as it may help with sleeping well and balance in life.

Lifestyle

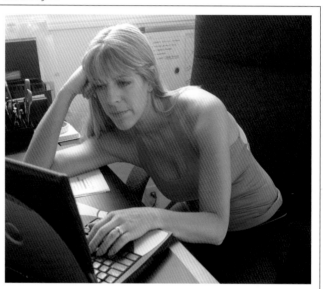

- If you work a job where you are required to walk a lot, you will burn more calories than someone who sits.

- If you go from a physically active job to a sedentary job, you might gain weight or have a harder time losing it.

- As we age, we generally move less. This is why the effects of aging are so common, because we lose bone and muscle when we do not use them.

ISOMETRIC TRAINING
Why holding a muscle can activate more of it

Earlier we covered the different types of muscle contractions: concentric, eccentric, and isometric. Isometric is a contraction that does not change the length of the muscle. Imagine doing a biceps curl and stopping halfway and holding it there—that is an isometric contraction. You can use this type of contraction at any range of motion for all muscles.

Many Pilates exercises for the abs utilize isometric contraction, as you move your arms and legs but keep your torso still. Isometric training is most common with ab work, but it is important to do for all muscles because of its ability to activate muscle fibers that are not commonly used. Think of isometric training as being like overloading your circuits—but not in a bad way.

Because we move in similar patterns in life and exercise, we often use the same muscle fibers over and over again. These fibers have become strong and easily connect to our brains

Isometric Biceps

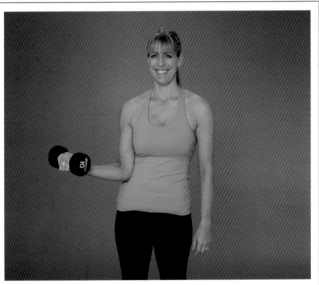

- Within a biceps curl, you have several points in the range of motion to create a safe isometric exercise.

- Make sure you stabilize your shoulder and elbow by using your back muscles to keep your shoulder back and down.

- Use an easy to moderate weight to start; you can always increase later.

- Start by holding for 30 to 45 seconds and gradually increase to 60 to 90 seconds.

Isometric Leg Lift

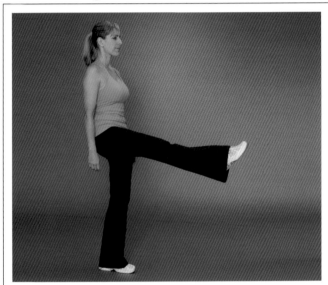

- Stand with your feet shoulder width apart to start.

- Lift one leg in the air with a locked knee and pointed toe. Hold your leg as high as you can for 60 seconds.

- Keep your abs engaged and make sure to keep breathing.

- This isometric exercise will work your standing hip and the quads and hip flexors of the leg you are holding.

when we need to move. But within each muscle are groups of fibers that do not need to work unless the movement patterns change or the load becomes so heavy that they have to help out.

Let's pretend that there are one hundred muscle fibers in your biceps, but you only ever use twenty of them. Using isometric training will recruit the fibers that are already available, the ones you use all the time, and then once they fatigue, your body will need to call on the other ones. So maybe now, after doing some isometric training for your biceps, you are able to contract and use fifty of the fibers. This example is not accurate science but it demonstrates how your brain and body use and recruit muscle fibers. Isometric training is a great way to "turn on" your muscles and maximize the use of what you have!

Isometric Abs

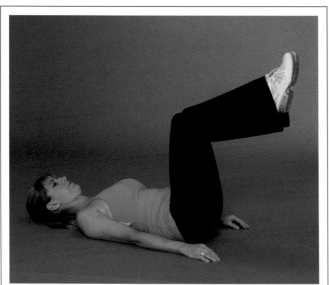

- Most of us are more connected to the abdominal fibers closest to the rib cage, because the most common ab exercises lift the upper body. Using isometrics to activate the lower body is very beneficial.

- Keep your ankles above your knees and start with the knees over your navel.

- Keep your lower back on the ground and try to relax your head and shoulders as well.

- Your abs will resist your legs from pulling your pelvis forward and off the ground.

Isometric Resistance

- Start off any isometric exercise with a moderate amount of resistance and hold for 30 to 45 seconds.

- In every range of motion for all joints, there are end points. Work somewhere in the middle or at the beginning of the range to build some strength first.

- Start with static resistance—constant unmoving resistance—before adding dynamic resistance, which is force that has movement to it.

- Isometric training is most effective when you use your brain to help activate the muscles.

WHICH MUSCLES?

Connecting to the muscles from your rib cage to pelvis

We concentrate on the rectus abdominis, obliques, and transversus abdominis when we do isometric exercises to strengthen the abs. Knowing where these muscles are can help you visualize them becoming shorter and contracting. I like to tell my clients to think of an accordion. Knowing that the muscles attach from the rib cage to the pelvis, visualize the rib cage moving closer to the pelvis like an accordion. In isometric training, you still want to visualize them moving closer together, even if you are not actually moving your bones or spine. You still fire the muscles and contract them, even if they are not actually shortening very much. The idea of an isometric contraction is that the muscle fibers want to move closer together but are being held at one length. This causes the brain to continue to send signals to the muscles to activate them. The rectus abdominis and obliques are external muscles that have similar attachments

Isometrics = Brain Power + Muscle

- Any time you do an isometric exercise, you want to be able to visualize what you are asking the muscle to do.

- Practicing isometrics can help increase the number of muscle fibers you use every day as well as in exercise.

- Isometric training involves a great deal of brain power as well as muscle. You will gain a new level of body control from doing isometrics.

Needle and Thread Motion

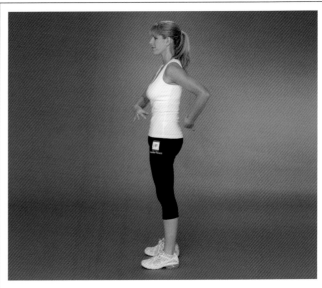

- Stand in an upright posture with your hips, rib cage, and neck aligned.

- Imagine a needle and thread in front of your navel.

- Thread it through your navel and pull it out of your back. Your abs should pull in toward your spine.

- Hold this position without moving your ribs, hips, or spine, and squeeze to make it harder. This will contract your transversus abdominis.

and direction. Using the accordion example can help activate these muscles easily.

The transversus abdominis is a deeper core muscle that works when you laugh or cough. In fact, it's a good idea to think about these motion to activate it. I also like to use what I call needle and thread visualization which is explained below. You can use this in any position, but it is easier to understand when explained in this position. Your brain is the messenger of the signal to contract. The more clear you are about where the signal is going, the more muscle fibers will be contracted and the more results you will experience.

Science can be fun when you apply it to your body. The more you know about how your body works, the more you can do to make it better!

Accordion Motion for Abs

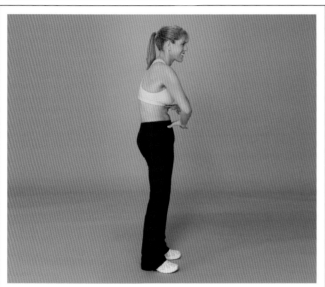

- Stand upright to learn this, but you can use it in any position and with any muscle so learning how to visualize this can help in other exercises, too.

- Imagine your rib cage and pelvis are the front and back end of an accordion and the muscles in between are what get squeezed to play the instrument.

- Imagine you are going to move both ends together without moving your spine.

- Concentrate on shortening them to engage them.

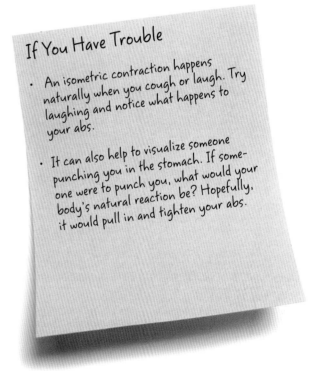

If You Have Trouble

- An isometric contraction happens naturally when you cough or laugh. Try laughing and notice what happens to your abs.

- It can also help to visualize someone punching you in the stomach. If someone were to punch you, what would your body's natural reaction be? Hopefully, it would pull in and tighten your abs.

WHEN TO DO THEM
How and when to use isometric exercises

Because isometric exercises are static—you don't move—you can literally do them anywhere! From sitting at your desk all day to using them in every exercise you do, isometric ab training is a great way to strengthen your core all day long. You can apply this training to other exercises and muscle groups, too, and because you can contract your abs without moving your body, most people will not even know that you are exercising! Doing an isometric squat at work might have

people wondering and could cause distraction, but doing abs can be your secret. Wherever you do them, make sure not to hold your breath. Just because you are squeezing and holding a muscle does not mean you hold your breath.

The trick is to learn how to use your brain to contract only these muscles and not get others involved. The more you practice, the better you will get at it and you will find greater ease in holding a contraction for 60 to 90 seconds without

In the Car

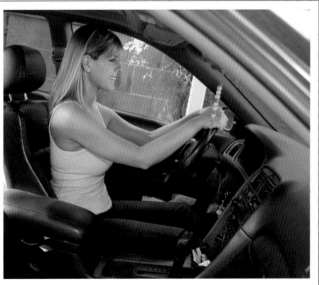

- Make sure you are upright and not leaning your back against the seat.

- Good posture is shoulders back and down and your spine erect, away from the seat.

- Imagine a needle and thread going through your belly button and pulling out the back.

- Also focus on pulling your rib cage together from left to right side and your pelvis the same way. Squeeze everything into the center of your body.

At Your Desk

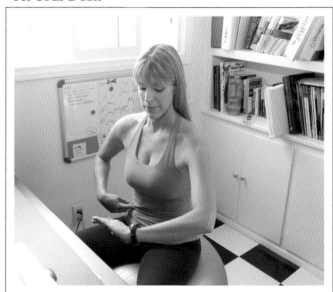

- With your feet flat on the ground and body upright, you can perform isometric abs at your desk.

- Do not allow your back to lean on the chair or your arms to hold you up on your desk.

- Watch the clock and time yourself for 60 seconds; remember to keep breathing naturally as you squeeze your ab muscles.

- Do several sets in a row and increase the time if it gets too easy.

having to hold your breath. You do not need any extra resistance to get benefits. Use the power of your mind to contract at a level you can sustain for 60 seconds. When that gets easier, contract harder or hold longer.

During Cardio

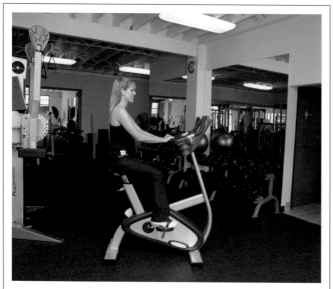

- It would actually be good form for you to use your abs in every exercise you do to stabilize your spine.

- In most cardio your body will do some bit of rotation or swaying, and keeping your abs tight can improve your form.

- Try using an isometric contraction when you do the hardest parts of your cardio workouts.

- Squeeze your abs for 60 to 90 seconds, throughout your cardio exercises.

During Other Exercises

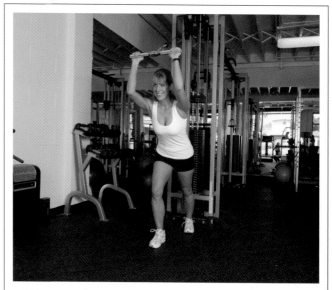

- Using your ab strength can make you stronger in any exercise you do.

- When you concentrate on squeezing your abs for the duration of each set of any exercise, you can also get a good ab workout.

- Focusing on your abs as well as the muscle group you are working on will help you focus your efforts where you need them.

- If you can concentrate on your abs in every exercise, you might not need any extra ab exercises in that workout session!

GETTING STARTED
The three best positions and progressions to use for isometric abdominal training

As you learn how to use your mind to contract your body, you might have a longer learning curve as you adapt to and feel confident about this method of training. Motion is sometimes easy to learn because you follow a pattern or can imitate what you see. Isometric training is invisible to the eye and controlled by the mind. Expect to start slowly if you are a beginner and be patient with the learning curve. If you have been an athlete, dancer, or martial artist in the past, you will have a much easier time, because you have had to learn how to control your body in other situations.

The partner exercise below is designed to be a testing tool for you to feel what is required of your body and as a way to

Seated with a Partner

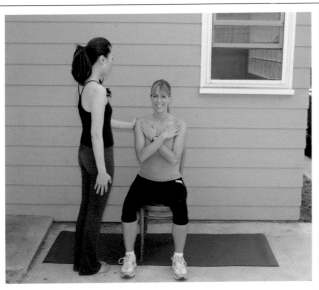

- Use this exercise to test your ab strength improvement every few weeks or months. You will need a partner.

- Sit on the edge of a chair or ledge with your feet flat and spine erect.

- Cross your arms over your chest and think of being a statue. Contract your abs isometrically and hold them as your partner gently challenges you in all directions.

- The partner should apply force slowly. Your challenge is to not move at all.

Supine Isometric Beginner

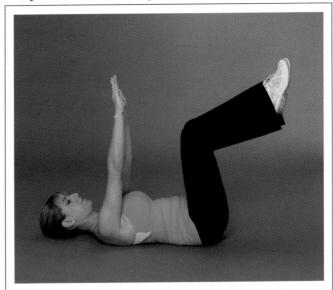

- On your back with the small of your back pressed into the ground, lift your arms up to the ceiling and legs to tabletop as shown in the image above.

- Resist the weight of your legs pulling your back off the floor and your pelvis forward. Resist the weight of your arms pulling your rib cage off the ground.

- Hold your arms and legs here for 45 to 60 seconds while isometrically contracting your abs.

get feedback about how well you are holding yourself as a statue. The supine exercise with your arms and legs can be broken up into parts: upper, lower, and both. The plank on your elbows is a more advanced exercise, but I encourage you to try it at least once to see what it is like and how well you do.

There are many, many more exercises you can do isometrically with similar motions. You can adjust and modify any of them to fit your body, fitness level, or goals. When using the seated with a partner exercise, know that you can progress to standing and seated on a ball for a more intense exercise. Tell your partner to use a light amount of force, hold each force for at least 5 seconds, and keep changing direction. A partner can offer resistance to forward and backward motion, side to side, and rotation.

Supine Isometric Intermediate

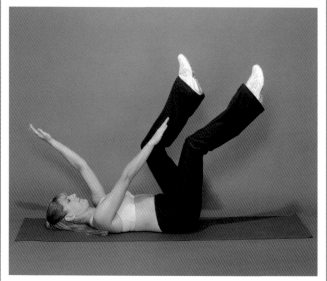

- To add more resistance to this position, start by very slowly moving your arms over your head one at a time like scissors, as you maintain contact with the floor and do not move your rib cage.

- Using your legs as resistance is often much harder because your legs weigh more than your arms.

- With knees bent, slowly scissor the arms and legs back and forth to add resistance as you maintain your core in touch with the floor.

Elbow Plank

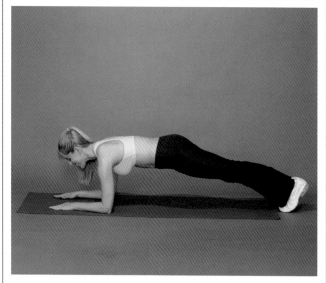

- Start by placing your elbows and forearms on the floor, shoulder width apart.

- Bring your knees to the floor and adjust your body-weight so most is on your arms. Depending on how much you weigh, this may be easy or very hard. You might want to use a pillow under your knees.

- Keep your abs contracted by pulling in and holding for 60 seconds.

- When this position gets easy, move from the knees onto the toes.

NEED MORE?

You can safely and effectively add extra resistance to isometric ab exercises

Adding more resistance to your body during exercise should be done safely and strategically. Just adding a weight to an exercise can increase the risk without increasing the benefit, so know what you are doing before you do it. I always encourage using body weight first before adding different forms of resistance, because you manage the use of your body weight on a daily basis. Practice adding more force from your own body weight first, because this gives you a resistance program you can take with you anywhere you go. There are a few isometric and Pilates mat exercises that demonstrate the progression of using your own body weight that I am going to demonstrate here.

Isometric with One Leg

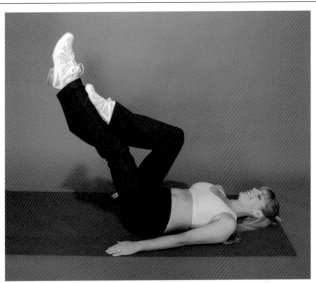

- Start by lying on the floor, legs in tabletop position.

- Keep your lower back on the ground and your abs engaged. Without lifting off the ground, extend one leg out in front of you while keeping the other leg bent.

- The extended leg adds more resistance to you trying to keep your lower back on the ground.

- Make sure you keep it at an angle that is challenging but comfortable. Switch legs each time you do it.

Isometric with Two Legs

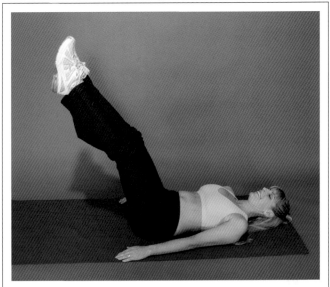

- Lie on the floor and extend both legs in front of you at a 45-degree angle or less. To make it easier, bring your legs up closer to you and toward the ceiling.

- This position offers double the intensity of the last exercise, so be sure to notice how your back feels. If you start to come off the ground, it is too intense.

- Hold for 60 seconds with your abs engaged and lower back on the ground.

Other forms of resistance that you can add to ab exercises include tubing, small free weights or ankle weights, cables, water, and vibration, such as the Bodyblade. In the exercises on this page, you use mainly your legs as resistance. The longer your legs, the harder it will be. I am using a 45-degree angle as your starting point, but you can bring the leg closer to your body (up and in) to make it easier on your abs and back. If you want to make it more difficult, you can lower the leg closer to the ground, but be sure to press your lower back into the floor at all times. If you cannot push your lower back into the floor, the resistance will be too much for you, and you might feel the resistance in your back.

Iso Abs, Moving Legs

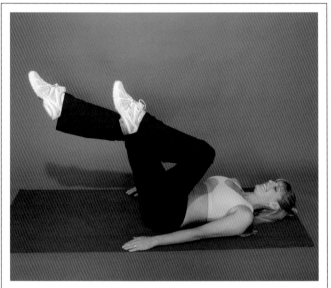

- This is a dynamic exercise where you hold your abs and torso still while moving only your legs.

- On your back with legs in tabletop to start, press your lower back into the ground. Move your legs back and forth from a bent-knee position to extended out in front of you, alternating sides.

- Take 2 counts or more to alternate from side to side. This should be done slowly with the focus on keeping the lower back on the ground.

Rules for Increasing Intensity

- Always test yourself with the least amount of resistance first to see how well you do. Repeat several times to make sure you'll be able to handle increased resistance.

- Use one leg at a time to add resistance. The closer your leg is to your body, the easier it is.

- Move farther away slowly to see how much your abs can handle.

- If you are moving all around, you are using too much intensity.

WHAT ARE CRUNCHES?

Learn the basics to get the most out of this exercise

The crunch is the most common ab exercise, replacing the once-popular full sit-up, where people used to anchor their feet under a bed or dresser to help them come all the way up from the floor to a seated position. A full sit-up uses your hip flexors at the end of the motion more than your abs, so we moved to concentrate on crunching, because it targets the abs better.

Hopefully by now you have learned a little bit more about your abs and have a clear picture in your mind about what should be moving when you work them. As I tell most clients and classes, the abs connect the rib cage and the pelvis, so these are the places you should move first. The abs do not connect to the neck, head, or arms, so concentrating on these will not help your abs do their job.

Like the example of the accordion, you should concentrate on pulling one half of your body toward the other or one

Half Crunch Upper, Start

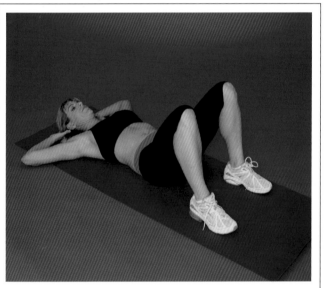

- You can put your hands behind your head, cross them over your chest, or extend them over your head for extra resistance.

- Keep your feet flat on the ground about hip width apart and knees bent.

- Think about moving the rib cage first. Try putting one hand on your rib cage to practice feeling the movement being initiated here.

- Inhale when you are on the ground and get ready to exhale as you lift yourself off the ground.

Half Crunch Upper, Finish

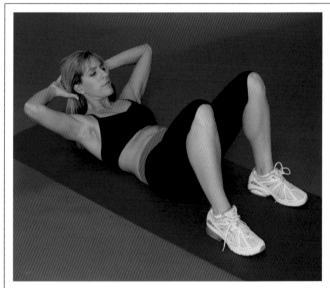

- Using your rib cage to move you, the upper portion of your abs should start to pull toward your navel.

- Once your rib cage is initiated and it's pulling you, your chest, shoulders, and head should also lift off the ground.

- Use 2 counts to bring yourself off the ground and exhale as you lift; inhale as you lower yourself back down using 2 counts to lower.

- Pull yourself as far up as you can using your abs.

half toward the center. Because you can move both sides independently, I divide crunches into half crunches so that you focus only on moving one half of your body. You should focus on moving from the place where the abs attach: the rib cage or pelvis.

I see too many people pulling on their necks or throwing themselves into this position, and they do not reap the benefits because of incorrect form. Depending on the length of their neck and spine, some people may feel this exercise in their necks no matter what because of their mechanics.

Adjust the exercise to fit your body, but for maximum benefit and less pressure on your neck, make sure to initiate the movement where the muscle is attached.

Half Crunch Lower, Start

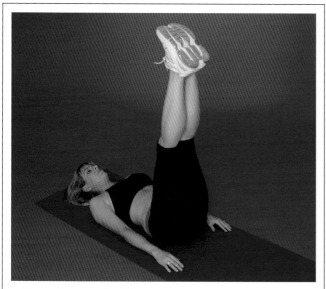

- Lie on the ground with legs in tabletop and head on the mat.

- Rest your arms at your sides and do not push them against the ground for help.

- Concentrate on the abs attached to your pelvis and the direction they will be pulling—in toward the center and your rib cage.

- Focus on not using your legs to help you. Maybe press your knees together to keep them still.

Half Crunch Lower, Mid-Range

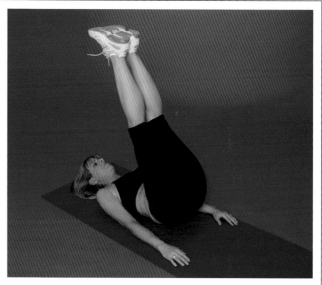

- Use the abs at your pelvis to pull your entire lower body in toward the center of your body.

- You will lift off the ground in an arc motion; it will be much harder than the half crunch upper.

- Exhale as you lift your lower body off the ground.

- If this is uncomfortable on your back in anyway, try adjusting your knees or legs to make it more comfortable. If it hurts, do not do it.

WHAT TO MOVE

You have two areas of your body to initiate a crunch

If you're like a lot of people, you learned how to do ab crunches from a video or in a class. In a class situation, you often have music to drive the speed of your motion—if you allow it to. The danger is that you sacrifice good form for speed and develop a bad habit.

As I have mentioned, the abs attach the rib cage to the pelvis and vice versa. Learning how to connect your brain to these physical places and have them move first may be a new concept for you. If this is the case, be patient with yourself and know that your crunches will bring you more results once you gain control over these parts of your body. Chances are that if you learn to pull yourself up with your abs, you will not experience the same stress on your neck as when you lift with your neck.

Core awareness can also help protect your back and joints because you are more aware of your body. When you know

Ribs

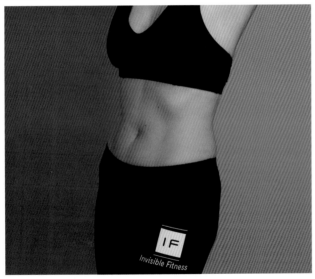

- The rib cage consists of a set of twelve ribs that creates a cage for your heart, lungs, and other organs.

- The big flat bone in the front of the rib cage that connects the two sides together is called the sternum.

- The ribs are connected to the spine in the thoracic area, which is the bottom of the neck to the lower back.

- The attachments for your rectus abdominis and obliques are along the rib cage from front to back.

Pelvis

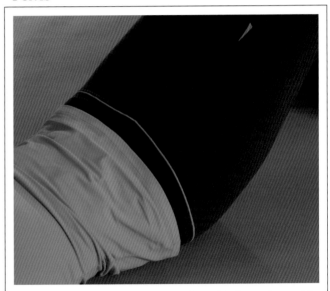

- A woman's pelvis is wider than a man's, due to her childbearing abilities.

- The pelvis acts as a protector for the sexual organs just like the rib cage protects other organs.

- The pelvic bone along with the femur makes up the hip joint.

- The pelvic bone is higher in the back and on the sides than in the front.

how to turn on your muscles, you can use them more often and effectively in all your activities and movements. There are more core muscles that we will not cover here, such as the quadratus lumboruem and the spinal erectors.

The Neck

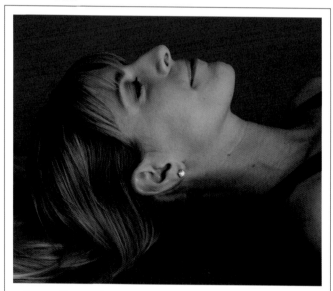

- Depending on the length of your neck and mobility of your spine, you may feel discomfort when performing some core exercises.

- Because your head weighs approximately 12 pounds, your neck muscles work to lift your head during crunches.

- If you can bend your neck and tuck your chin, you will decrease the amount of work for your neck.

- If you feel a general tightness and no serious discomfort, remember that your muscles are working.

Understanding Your Anatomy

- Knowing anatomy can help you determine if you are experiencing the right things in an exercise.

- If you feel your neck or lower back more than your abs, the exercise is either too advanced for you at this point or not appropriate for your structure.

- Understanding where things attach and what joints they cross help you to determine if you are moving from the right place.

CRUNCHES

FORM & THOUGHT
How you do a crunch can determine how effective it will be

Now that you know where all your muscles are, we have to talk about how to use them, what you might be feeling, and what muscles you may want to stop using. You know by now that the brain has to send a message to the muscles to get them to "turn on." You want to be aware of what you are supposed to be moving to make sure the right bones and muscles move first for optimal contraction. Does this mean you will always have to spend time thinking about your exercise

before and as you do it? Yes. But if you are a beginner or have been doing "brainless" exercise for some time, once you practice using your brain to control your body with conscious awareness, it gets easier and more natural as time goes on.

I once had a client tell me she wanted me to fix her posture. She wanted me to strengthen her body so she would not have to think about standing up straight ever again. I gently informed her that getting to that point was nearly impossible

Hip Flexors

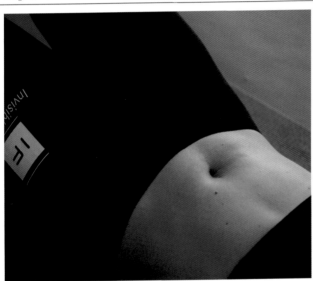

- The hip flexors are made up of three muscles: psoas major, psoas minor, and iliacus.

- The hip flexors connect the lower back and pelvis to the femur (thigh bone).

- While we can't turn the hip flexors off in ab exercises, we don't want them to dominate the movement.

- Squeezing a pillow or ball between your legs can help you focus on using the ab muscles more than the hip flexors during crunches.

The Lower Back

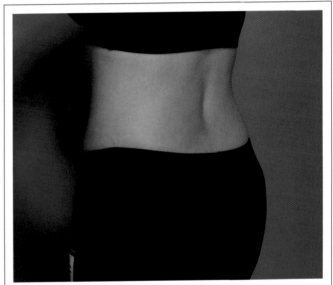

- Many people have soreness or tightness in the lower back due to sitting all day or because of a tilted pelvis.

- When doing ab exercises, concentrate on moving the abs so the brain can disconnect from the back and it can release the lower back from any tension.

- If you normally have an anterior tilt of the pelvis, your lower back is in a contraction all day.

- Doing abdominal work can help to actively stretch the back and release tension.

(without a brace!). I explained how the brain has to tell the muscles what to do and that she would have to learn how to stand up straight by thinking about it.

Once you practice good posture, it becomes second nature. I may sit or slouch sometimes because I am tired, but I have trained myself to stand or sit with good posture to the point that if I am slouching for long, my body lets me know! When you practice anything, it gets easier. Give yourself some time to use the information and new ways of thinking presented in this book to build a new relationship with your body.

Your Middle

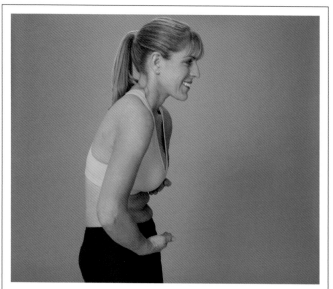

- Remember that your abs attach your rib cage to your pelvis.

- When you want to use your abs to either support you with an isometric contraction or move you with a concentric contraction, moving from your middle first will help you engage the right muscles.

- Whether you are in a class or working out on your own, you control your body. For optimal performance and results, always be mindful and inquisitive about what you should be feeling, thinking, and moving.

What to Think About

- If you have used your hips and lower back in your ab exercises in the past, do not focus on them now.

- When you think about a muscle, your brain talks to it and engages it even just a little. Thinking about a muscle will turn it on, and we want to turn off the lower back and hip muscles.

- As you exercise, imagine all the muscles you have learned about and what they look and feel like as they contract.

SPEED & INTENSITY

Know how to use these properly for safe and effective workouts

When starting an exercise program, you must consider all your goals and choose exercises and ways to do the exercises that support you achieving those goals. We talked about doing crunches in an exercise class situation, where the beat of the music drives your rep speed at the possible detriment of good form. How fast or slow should you go?

Exercise physiology tells us that applied force over a certain duration of time produces a result specific to the time under tension. If you do something quickly with explosive force, you train your body to activate a large group of muscles quickly and for a very short duration. These same muscles would not necessarily be as good with large amounts of force for an extended period of time.

There is a principle in exercise called the SAID principle: specific adaptation for imposed demand. Simply put, if you only do biceps curls, you will only build your biceps. If you

Muscle Building—Large Weights

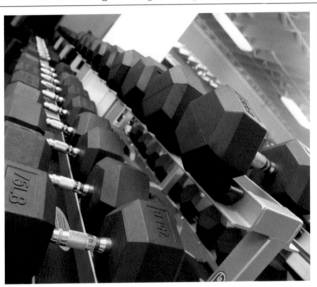

- If you want to build muscles to increase your metabolism, there are guidelines for speed and intensity.

- Aim for 2-3 sets per exercise, one to two exercises per muscle group, and a rep speed of 6 seconds each, totaling 60 seconds of constant work.

- You want to choose an intensity that pushes you close to failure at the end of the 60 seconds.

- Take a 60-second rest between each set and exercise if possible.

Explosive Strength—Power Lifting

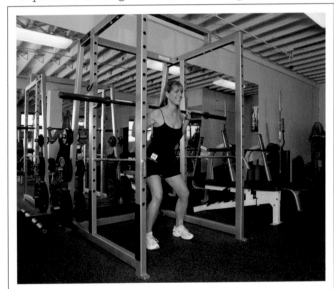

- Explosive strength calls for increased intensity and speed.

- This is more of a mental exercise initially because you need to send a specific and powerful brain "charge" to as many muscle fibers in the muscles you want to use very quickly.

- Choose an intensity level of 9 on a scale of 1 to 10. This is a higher risk exercise because of the speed, so start slowly and work your way up to more intense resistance and speed.

only walk on the treadmill, you will only increase your ability to walk on the treadmill. That ability will not translate to being better at cycling or swimming.

When choosing how fast and intense your exercises should be, keep several factors in mind. What is your goal? What is the best form and speed to reach that goal and why? For instance, when doing a muscle-building program, physiology shows us that constant tension on a muscle for about 60 seconds is what stimulates the most effective hypertrophy (muscle building). This goal also requires that you do enough sets to take your muscle to failure. I recommend a 6-count rep speed for this goal.

When it comes to speed, start slowly. Learn control over your movement and body and only increase your speed once you have complete control.

Sprinting

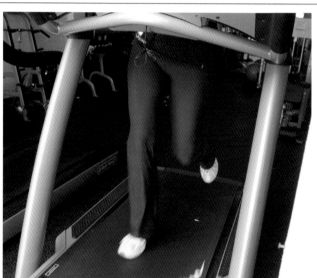

- Training for a marathon and training for a sprint are different in how you use speed and intensity.

- When you increase intensity by doing something very fast, the body has to recruit more muscle and work harder.

- Make sure your body can handle running for 15 or 20 minutes straight before increasing the intensity and speed for an explosive 3 or 5 minutes.

- Build a foundation in your ankles, hips, and abs before increasing intensity.

Ab Training

- The reason you may need speed in your core is usually related to some kind of cardio.

- To achieve optimal performance in training, I recommend that you always start slowly and gain control and strength of your muscles before increasing speed and intensity.

- One of my educators liked to say, "Own it before you load it," and I completely agree!

- Follow the 4- to 6-second rep speed model when starting, and gradually increase the intensity and then speed to suit your goals.

111

CHOOSING VOLUME

How many crunches and how often depends on your goals and current fitness level

Some people like to do hundreds of crunches every day. It helps them to focus on the number, the burn, and the results they have obtained in the past. Doing fewer crunches might make them nervous that they aren't doing enough. But do you need to do hundreds of crunches each day? Not necessarily. But again it depends on your goals. Not everyone has the same goal, so you should train according to the outcome you desire, along with a basic understanding of the results you can expect from the exercises and form you choose.

If you're a beginner who has been sedentary for months or even years, I recommend setting a goal of a short duration of time and consistency. If you have not worked out at all, and

Logging Workouts

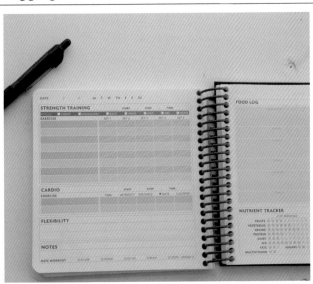

- If you are a beginner, consider keeping a journal or creating an exercise spreadsheet.

- Many people wait until they "have time to exercise," which leads them to not exercise at all. Schedule it in your calendar like you would dinner with friends.

- Log your workouts to gauge how it is working over time.

- Adjust your volume based on your results. Every program will need to progress to the next level in order for you to continue seeing results.

How Many Exercises?

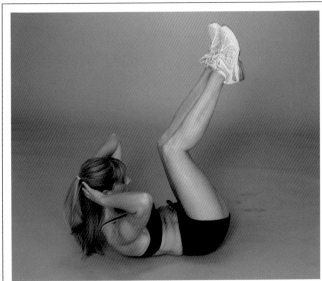

- If you're a beginner, start out with one exercise at a time and learn the correct form.

- Work out at an intensity level until you feel fatigued; see if you notice those muscles a day or two later.

- If you're an intermediate exerciser, you may need two or three different exercises per workout.

- If you're an advanced exerciser, three to four exercises are all you really need to fatigue your abs. If this is not enough, increase the intensity level.

you want to start working on your abs, setting a goal to exercise 6 or 7 days a week might be unrealistic. You don't want to set yourself up to fail. Set smaller goals and allow yourself to succeed at accomplishing them consistently. Aim to work out 3 to 4 days a week for maybe 15 to 20 minutes each time. Once you can do that for 3 to 4 weeks, increase one element of your program.

If you're an advanced exerciser and already work out 1 hour, 4 or 5 days a week, you may want to adjust your form, slow down your movement, and not change anything else. The great thing about creating your own exercise program is that you can design it to fit your life and your goals. Most people do not stick to certain programs because there are too many obstacles to overcome. There is no absolute amount of exercise that has to be done, so you can have full control over how much and how often you exercise.

How Many Reps?

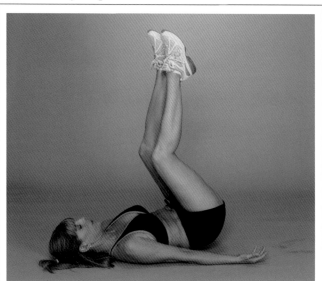

- If you are a beginner, you want to aim for about 90 seconds per set.

- Your rep speed will determine how many you need to do to reach the 90-second mark. Start with 4-second reps, which should equal 20 to 25 crunches.

- If you are an intermediate or advanced exerciser, increase your intensity and slow down the movement.

- Aim for 60 seconds of constant work at a 6-second rep speed. Try 10 to15 reps very slowly.

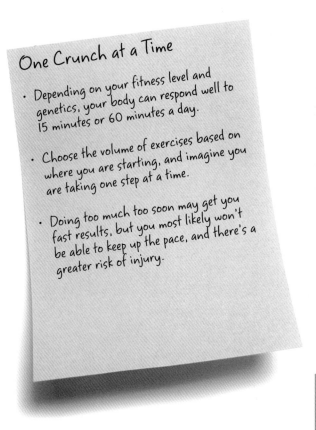

One Crunch at a Time

- Depending on your fitness level and genetics, your body can respond well to 15 minutes or 60 minutes a day.

- Choose the volume of exercises based on where you are starting, and imagine you are taking one step at a time.

- Doing too much too soon may get you fast results, but you most likely won't be able to keep up the pace, and there's a greater risk of injury.

113

WHAT DOES IT WORK?

The bicycle exercise works your abs differently than a crunch

Another popular ab exercise is the bicycle. This exercise incorporates rotation as well as flexion of the spine, so it uses the obliques more than—or at least as much as—a crunch. Next to the crunch, I see people doing this exercise most in their ab routines.

On these pages I will review the form and different variations of difficulty for each level of exerciser. Know that you can always make an exercise easier or harder, depending on your goal. If you are a beginner, keeping your legs up in the air might be too intense for you to think about doing the motion properly, because you are trying really hard just to keep the starting form. I am going to outline three variations of this exercise, and even if you're the most advanced exerciser, I encourage you to do the beginner's version a few times to practice moving from your ribs first, not your head, neck, or shoulders. I also urge you to do the beginner version

A Locked Spine = Not Good

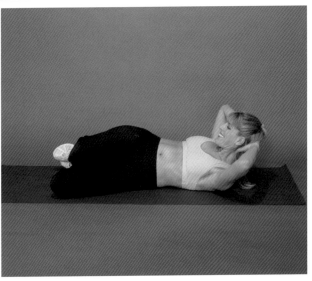

- This exercise can be dangerous due to several factors related to your active versus passive range of motion.

- Because the weight of your legs can pull you into a range of motion your body does not have, this could cause injury.

- If you have any back problems, don't do this exercise; it may increase your risk for pain.

- If you do not want to move both sides of your body, you can keep a neutral position.

Neutral Position, Start

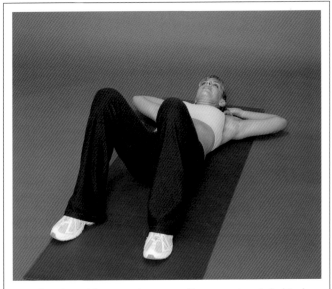

- Rather than risk your spine and back problems, you can use a neutral start position if you only want to move the top half of your body.

- Your feet should be flat on the ground, hip width apart, and your lower back should be in contact with the floor.

- Place your hands behind your head so you focus on moving from the ribs and don't get distracted by your neck.

- Inhale before you move and exhale as you initiate and execute the movement.

with your eyes closed, so you can visualize the abs pulling your rib cage up and over like a pulley, and then also visualize the abs attached to the opposite hip pulling in toward the center to meet the rib cage.

As we look at the body more closely on the next few pages, please be aware of spinal rotation. Every part of the spine has a different amount of rotation, so this action should never be forced. Locking one half of the body in an extreme range of motion while trying to rotate the other side can lead to injury. Make sure your motions do not cause discomfort in your spine.

Mid-Range Position

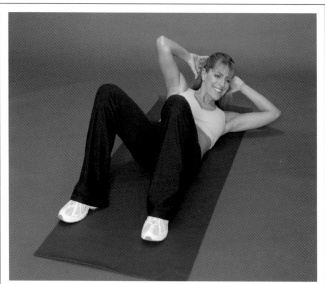

- Pull your upper body from the rib cage first in a diagonal direction.

- Depending on your body type and structure, you may not have a large range of motion in this position.

- Use your brain to connect to the muscle fibers attached along the ribs and move these first.

- Exhale as you come up slowly for 2 counts and then gently lower back down and inhale.

Everyone Is Built Differently

- You can take any exercise and modify it to fit your body, as well as make it easier or harder.

- Each section of the spine has a different degree of rotation available.

- The most important part of this exercise is moving from the muscles you want to use and visualizing them contracting.

- Your range of motion is determined by your structure. You can add mechanisms and tools to the exercise to create more motion later.

USING THE RIGHT MUSCLES
Knowing which muscles to fire first helps you activate them

In this exercise you will use the major core muscles, but you will focus on your obliques first and rectus abdominis second. When you think about doing the exercise, you will again initiate the movement from your rib cage, but instead of pulling down like an accordion toward your pelvis—the way you would for a crunch—you will pull the rib cage toward the opposite hip. Many trainers and instructors cue elbow to opposite knee to give you an idea of the direction you

want to move, but the abs do not attach to the elbows or the knees. Instead, you should practice initiating the movement from your ribs and focus on that diagonal, pulling toward your pelvis on the opposite side.

When dealing with your active rotation, you may want to gently test how far you can comfortably twist in each direction. Do not throw your body or push it into rotation; allow your muscles to pull you there. You may find, based on your

Twisting to the Left

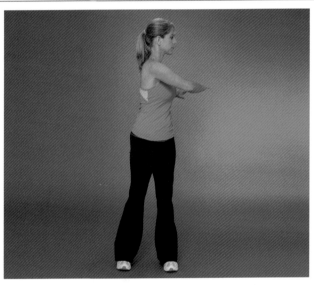

- Test your active range of motion first to find out how far you can rotate comfortably in each direction.

- Make a note of any imbalance or pain you experience from side to side.

- Pay attention to how your body feels and any signs it may be giving you.

- Do not force more range of motion than you have comfortably. You are testing your active, pain-free range of motion.

Obliques to the Rib Cage

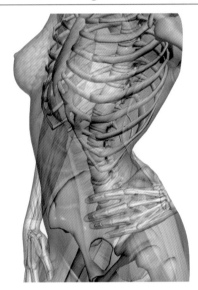

- When you rotate or twist, visualize the bottom of the lower ribs initiating the motion and pulling your body off the ground.

- Your obliques are under your rectus abdominis and can perform spinal flexion as well as rotation.

- These muscles are always working when you move; you really cannot isolate them.

- Imagine that these muscles make up an invisible weight belt or support belt around your body to protect your spine.

structure and any previous conditions or injuries, that you have more range of motion on one side versus the other. This is actually quite common.

If you have pain when twisting, you might consider seeing a chiropractor to help align your spine and adjust your hips. Most doctors do not deal with bone issues beyond analyzing X-rays and prescribing antiinflammatories. You could also consult with a physical therapist or try acupuncture to alleviate inflammation and discomfort.

The goal for all exercise should be to work in a pain-free range of motion. When you add new exercises and movements, you may uncover some discomfort that you did not know was there. While you seek treatment and solutions for any pain, exercise in a pain-free range of motion only with control and conscious awareness.

Spine in Rotation

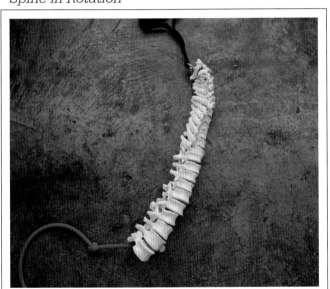

- The spine has thirty-three vertebrae, which are divided into three major sections. You also have fused bones under the lumbar called the sacrum and coccyx.

- The cervical spine consists of seven neck bones. They provide the most amount of rotation.

- The thoracic spine is made up of twelve vertebrae in the middle back. The lumbar spine has five vertebrae that make up the lower back. These have the least amount of rotation.

Use Your Own Body as a Guide

- Since the spine holds the spinal cord, which controls most of the body's functions, you want to be cautious when doing exercises centered on spinal movement.

- Because each person is built a little differently in terms of length of bones, joints, and muscles, your body may not be able to do exercises exactly like those around you can.

- Seek a professional to help you with any pain or discomfort you may discover or encounter when exercising.

HALF-BICYCLE

Doing a half-bicycle will help train your brain to lift from your rib cage

Most of us get so excited about starting a new exercise program that we do too much too soon and skip some important steps along the way. Also, when we've done the same thing over and over again, we often stop thinking about it and simply go through the motions. I recommend this exercise as a way to test your mind-body connection.

You might want to place your hand on your rib cage to sense whether or not this is the first thing that moves. If you don't feel your ribs move toward your midsection, you should not lift your head or shoulders off the ground. You can perform this exercise without doing it properly and get results, but you may use your neck more than you need to

Half-Bicycle, Start

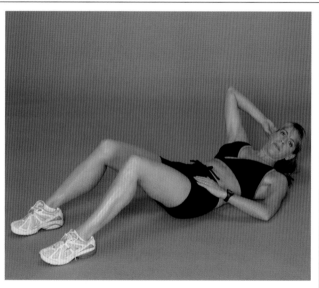

- Lie on the floor with your knees bent, feet flat, and hands behind your head.

- Close your eyes and get in touch with your rib cage and abs by visualizing them and where they are and connect in your body.

- Visualize the sensation of pulling from that place first and having your rib cage pull your upper body off the ground.

- Inhale to start and exhale as you contract and lift your upper body off the floor.

Half-Bicycle, Left Side

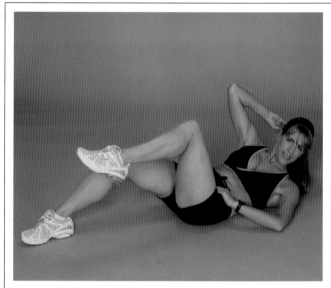

- Pull your upper body off the floor in an arc motion, toward the opposite hip.

- You can aim to bring your right elbow to your left knee for direction of motion, but remember to engage the muscles to pull you there.

- Exhale as you contract. Perform the motion slowly with 2 or 3 counts up and 2 or 3 counts down.

- Don't rest too long; immediately get in touch with the opposite side and execute another repetition on the other side.

which may cause strain in the neck. Good form is about using your brain first, having control, connecting to the right muscles, and moving in a way that is safe and effective for your muscles without unnecessary wear and tear on your joints. I like to use the half-bicycle with intermediate exercisers as a form of "brain training."

It's wise to start with the half-bicycle before moving onto the full bicycle because you have less resistance to deal with. You can really concentrate on initiating the motion from the appropriate muscles. When you skip ahead to the bicycle, the weight of your legs can distract you from maximizing the use of your brain. The resistance is greater, so your main concern is holding your body together against resistance, not necessarily doing it correctly.

Start off with a set or two of 30 slow reps and see how it goes. Because you count each side as 1 rep, you can increase the number of reps to get to fatigue before increasing the amount of sets.

Half-Bicycle, Right Side

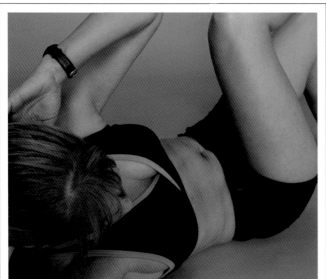

- You may or may not have the same available range of motion on both sides.

- If this is the case, do not pull or force yourself to do more on the limited side.

- Honor the controlled range of motion you have. You can seek to balance out your bones and musculature over time to help correct it through other alternative medical practices and exercise.

- For optimal results, use a constant slow and controlled motion.

Creating the Foundation First

- The half-bicycle is a great exercise for beginners to create a habit of using good form before making the exercise harder.

- This exercise allows advanced exercisers to test whether or not they pull from the right places.

- It also allows you to concentrate on your form without having to hold your lower body in the air.

- I use this exercise for all levels of exercisers to periodically test how well their brains are connected to their abs.

COMMON BICYCLE FORM

Once you establish the foundation, you can boost the intensity to increase results

After the half-bicycle becomes easy, it's time to graduate to the most common form of this exercise, which uses both sides of the body at a more intense level. I encourage you to reevaluate your form if you already include this exercise in your workout plan. I see people throw their bodies around with no control, and they do not have the strength or stamina

to do too many either. You can actually get more benefit from an exercise when you do fewer reps using proper form than doing more reps using incorrect form.

In the half-bicycle, you use both parts of your body, upper and lower, but you only have to lift one half of your body off the ground. Make sure you can hold your legs in tabletop

Bicycle, Start

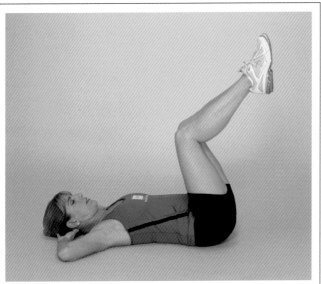

- Lie on your back on the floor; place your hands behind your head to support your neck.

- Make sure your hands do not pull on your neck. Keep your legs together and ankles above your knees—this will help reduce rotational inertia at the knee

and relieve pressure on your back.

- Keep you knees at a 45-degree angle and bring them closer to you to start. You can extend your legs farther away from your midsection to make it harder later.

Bicycle, Left Side

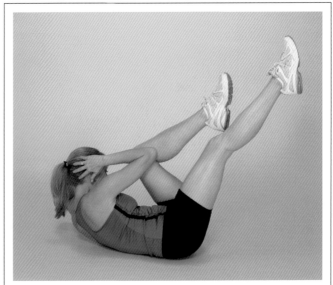

- Initiating from the rib cage, pull your upper body up and over toward your right knee.

- Using your hip and abs, draw in your left knee to meet your right elbow and upper body in the middle.

- If you have a long torso and short arms, you may not be able to touch your elbow to your knee and that is perfectly fine.

- The focus of the exercise is to bring both sides of your body into the center using your abs.

120

position for 45 to 60 seconds before adding more motion.

With this exercise, the increase in intensity for your abs is great, especially if you have long or large legs. Most of us do not practice exercises that build strength in the lower half of the abs, which makes resisting your legs easy. Most people only move the upper body, so they lack the strength and connection at the pelvis.

Bicycle, Mid-Range

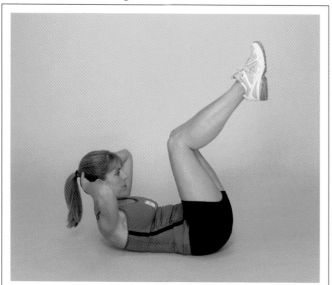

- As you change directions from the left to right, you have two options.

- You can lower back down to the ground to prepare to lift to the other side.

- Or you can stay in the middle in an isometric contraction to maximize your time. This is more difficult.

- When you pass through the middle on the way to the other side, visualize your abs—not your head or shoulders—moving your body.

Bicycle, Right Side

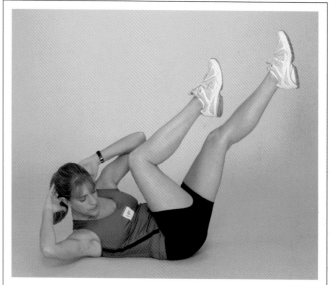

- After passing through the middle, switch gears to pull your torso to the right side.

- Using your right side to pull your torso up and in as your left knee helps guide your hips and abs into the center, extend your right leg.

- When doing the bicycle, the leg that is not bent and coming into the center can be extended at a 45-degree angle.

- The extended leg also acts as resistance to this exercise.

ADVANCED BICYCLE
Using your body weight in a different motion can add more resistance

When I work with someone who has made great progress and can handle intense exercises, I try to build on that foundation and make an exercise even harder before adding equipment or tools. I created this exercise out of the need for a more advanced version of the bicycle. I am sure there are many other versions that are good, too.

The first question to ask when you want to make an exercise harder is, "What is the easiest way to add more resistance with what I am already doing?" In the case of the bicycle, I assessed that from side to side we use only one extended leg for resistance. So I decided to add the other leg to increase the resistance. And since only half of the body pulls in one

Advanced Bicycle, Start

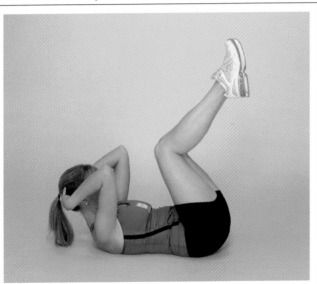

- Start this bicycle just as you would a regular bicycle, with legs in tabletop position.

- Keep your ankles above your knees and squeeze your legs together. They will move together, not separately.

- You can place your hands behind your head to start, but be careful not to pull on your neck.

- You will move your entire upper body to one side while you move your entire lower body to the other side.

Advanced Bicycle, Left Side

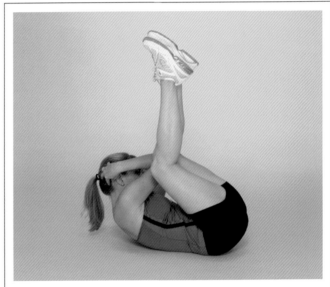

- Drawing both sides in from the middle, use your rib cage and pelvis to pull your upper and lower body close together.

- Pull your upper body toward the left and your lower body to the right.

- Take 2 counts to slowly pull both sides into the center.

- Exhale as you contract your abs and flex your spine.

direction, to increase the intensity I chose to have both sides of the body pull at the same time. Coordination, balance, and strength all get challenged in a motion in which you have already built strength by practicing the first two versions of this exercise. As in the regular bicycle, in this advanced version there is constant motion with no rest. You will hold your body off the floor while moving your limbs.

Advanced Bicycle, Mid-Range

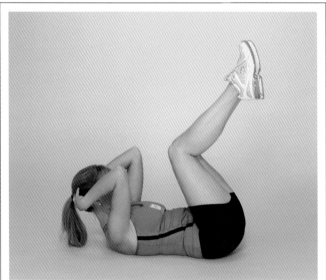

- To keep your balance and stability, come back to center; have your upper body hold a crunch off the ground.

- Inhale as you return to center; take a count or two before pulling to the other side.

- Because the center is not a rest position, your abs still hold an isometric contraction.

- Go slowly between each phase—left, middle, and side—so you can execute this with control.

Progression for the Advanced

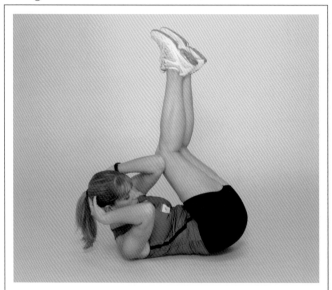

- This is an advanced exercise that should be added after a regular bicycle gets easy.

- To add even more resistance, extend your arms over your head instead of placing them behind your head.

- Extending your arms makes your upper body longer, hence the added resistance.

- There is no rest in this exercise until you stop the motion. If you need to rest before 45 to 60 seconds is up, this might be too difficult for you.

HOW MANY & HOW OFTEN

When it comes to ab work, quality is often more important than quantity

There is a myth that I want to debunk. It's called "toning." Toning as a verb in exercise does not exist. You burn calories, build muscle, or increase stamina—that is it. There is "tone" to your muscle, which means that your brain and nervous system are connected to it. When people experience nerve damage, the blood supply to the muscle is cut off and then there is

no tone. Most women believe that if they lift heavy weights, they will get big muscles. This is not true. Most women do not have enough testosterone to build big muscles like the bodybuilders you may have seen. Many women who engage in bodybuilding also take supplements and sometimes steroids to build big muscles. If you think lifting weights will

Muscle

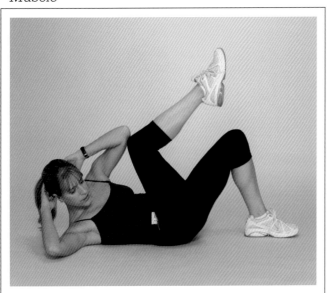

Strength

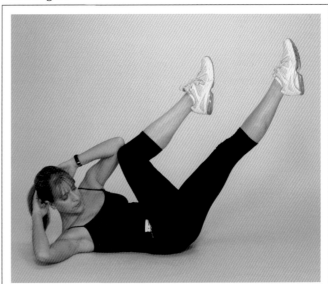

- When you want to build muscle, you have to use a force that is great enough to bring you to failure.

- Once the exercise becomes easier, you will have to increase the resistance to keep building.

- The abs do not build the same way some of the other surface muscles do because of the design and make up of the muscle.

- You can build muscle in your abs, but you may quickly reach your genetic limitation compared to the rest of your body.

- How you define strength will determine how you should train to build strength.

- Using your abs to support your body under extremely heavy loads should start with building muscle first.

- If you need ab strength that

is static or unmoving, doing isometric exercises and holding contractions for 1 to 2 minutes might be the way to train.

- If you need ab strength that is dynamic or moving, Pilates with a very heavy load might be the way to train.

124

make you look like these women, so you avoid resistance training, please think again. Resistance training can increase your metabolism and really impact your weight loss.

I've also heard women say that if they do many reps with light weights, they will just "tone" instead of "build" muscle. This also is not true. If your muscle is strong enough to lift 5 pounds 50 to 100 times, there is no reason for your body to change. Those 50 to 100 reps are simply a form of cardio for that muscle, because you don't build any muscle.

If you apply force to a muscle, you want a response. If the weight is heavy enough for you, you will build strength and muscle. If the weight offers a low level of resistance, you may build stamina if you lift it for a longer duration. What do you want to have happen with your abs? Are you looking to build stamina, strength, or muscle?

Stamina

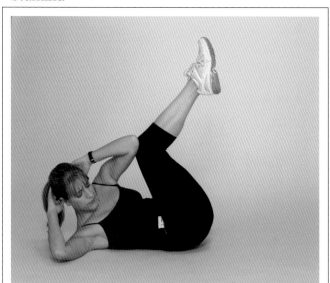

- We often need our core to hold us up all day at work.

- If you want to build stamina to play a sport, building some muscle and then doing the sport could be the most appropriate way to train.

- You could also take any ab exercise and do it for 5 to 10 minutes. Practice using your abs in your cardio and when you sit at your desk. This is a fast way to increase stamina for simple life activities.

How to Build Your Program

- Deciding on how many exercises, which ones, and how much resistance all depend on your goals.

- Change up your program at least every 6 months to continue to get results.

- If you've been using resistance to build muscle, try some exercises for stamina, and vice versa.

- Always use good form first, be connected to your body through your mind, and honor your body's current fitness level, range of motion, and limitations.

STABILITY TRAINING
Using unstable surfaces activates your abs to hold you together

You know the feeling you get when you start to lose your balance but catch yourself? Your whole body works to recover when you lose your balance like this, and hopefully you don't injure anything when it happens. But that feeling of intensity you get in your muscles is what you can learn to control and train in a safe and effective way to increase your ability to recover from a loss of balance as well as decrease the odds that you will need to.

When you stand on firm ground, you are stable, and if your body is aligned, a lot of your muscles are not really working too hard, as you are balanced over your joints. When you add instability under your feet, all of a sudden many of your muscles have to turn on and work to keep you from falling over or losing your balance.

Balance training is very popular these days, but it is not always safe. One of my pet peeves is trainers who have their

The Tree

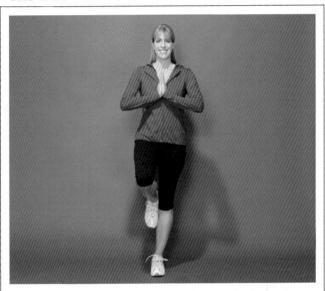

- Test your balancing ability with the tree.

- It's simple enough but shows whether or not someone can balance on one leg for 60 to 90 seconds. Start with your feet hip width apart and then transfer all your body weight to one leg.

- Lift your other leg and place your foot near the standing leg's ankle. Hold the other leg higher for more intensity. See if you can balance for 60 to 90 seconds on each leg.

Balance Board

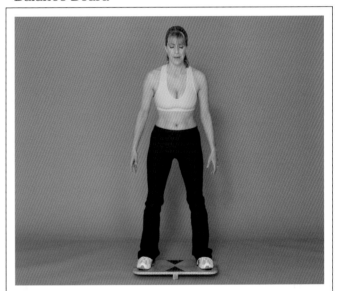

- There are many different kinds of boards and equipment built for challenging your stability.

- This is one of the easiest boards to use. Step on the board with one foot and then the other. You can rock gently side to side to start

until you can balance in the middle.

- Start by finding your balance in the middle; hold for 60 to 90 seconds. You can also do squats and other movement patterns to train your stability as you get stronger.

sedentary or beginner clients try to balance on an unstable surface and move their lower bodies while trying to do something with their upper bodies. This can lead to injury. Own it first before you load it, and don't ask your body to do too many things at once when you probably cannot do just one of those things well.

A safer way to use stability is through progression. Take one step at a time until it starts to become easier, and then add an exercise or more intensity to make it harder. Stability training can help to engage more of your core muscles and train them differently. This is a great way to add diversity with different benefits into your ab program.

Ball

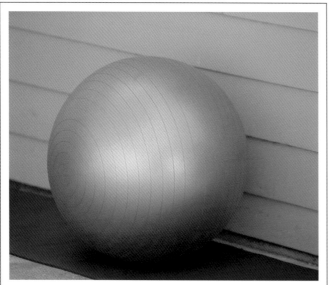

- There many types and sizes of balls out there, and they all have multiple functions.

- I use a ball to challenge stability for some exercises, to enhance resistance in others, and as a prop for exercise as well.

- Before buying a ball, decide what you want to do with it and read the instructions. The size of the ball may be important.

Practicing Stabilization

- When adding stability training to your program, start with the tree and see how well you do before adding harder exercises.

- Having a ball, balance board, or other tools can make it fun to practice your balance.

- Your core muscles hold you together. Challenging that will increase the stamina and strength of your core.

- Adding the ball to specifically challenge your core will also increase your results.

THE BALL AS A PROP
Exercises that use the ball to enhance the exercise

Sometimes using a prop can help you to focus differently when you do an exercise. When I started having people hold the ball or focus on moving the ball instead of moving themselves, the exercise motion would often improve.

You can add the ball as a prop to any exercise where you might not need your arms to support your head, or you can use your legs to hold the ball. Squeezing the ball between your legs can activate your adductors, otherwise known as

your inner thigh muscles, as well as increase the intensity of an exercise.

If you have a short neck or high shoulders, using your arms to hold the ball and moving your upper body can put more resistance on your neck than you are comfortable with. Try a few repetitions and see how you feel. Practice lifting from your rib cage and torso first to reduce the amount of work for your neck. If your body and neck keep engaging and you

Crunch with Ball, Start

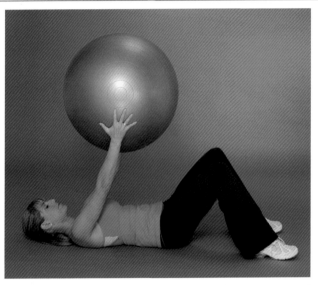

- With your feet flat on the ground and knees bent, hold the ball in your arms extended out in front of you.

- If the ball is too big for you, use a pillow instead.

- Inhale before you move and move from the rib cage first like in all other ab exercises.

- Even though you have added a prop, continue to use your brain to connect to the muscle you are using to initiate the motion.

Crunch with Ball, Finish

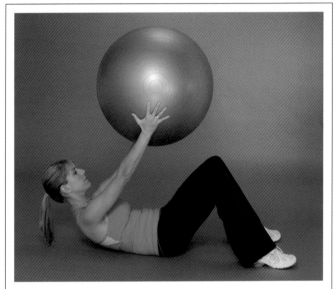

- With your arms extended, focus on placing the ball over your knees.

- Do not use momentum and "throw" your body forward; lift from your ribs and let your abs pull you up.

- Concentrate on the arc of motion that your spine and abs make as you move the ball up and over your knees.

- The amount of flexion you can achieve will depend on your spine. We will talk later about how to increase your range of motion, as explained on page 132.

still feel discomfort, you might need your hands to support your head.

Remember: Each of us is built differently. If you can't do a particular exercise, it's not necessarily the form or exercise that's the problem. It may be the fact that your body is not built to move that way. Honor your own unique structure and find exercises that best fit your body. Avoid blaming yourself or thinking that you are just weak or uncoordinated. Improving your body starts with some self-care, not negative self-talk.

Try these exercises and pay attention to what you feel in your body to see if they are good alternatives to an exercises you are currently doing. Also, if you use the ball as a prop, you can use something else in place of the ball such as a pillow or chair cushion.

Legs in the Air, Start

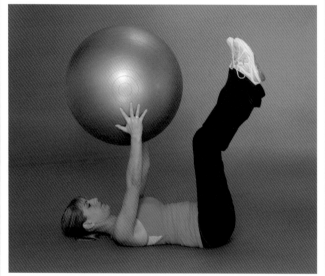

- To make a crunch with a ball more difficult, hold your legs in the air.

- This changes the angle you lift the ball and increases the degree of work on your lower body.

- You do not need to lock your knees, especially if you have long legs and it causes discomfort for your lower back.

- Keep your legs as straight as is comfortable and keep your legs tightly together.

Legs in the Air, Finish

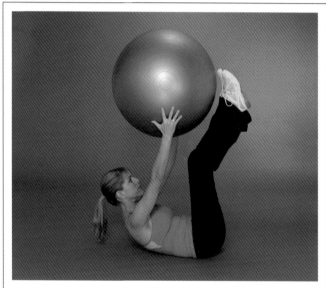

- The motion you make now is angled up at your feet versus over your knees.

- Lift your torso up with your abs first and aim to touch your feet with the ball.

- It's not important to actually touch the ball, but pretend you can so as to use your full range of motion.

- Exhale as you lift and take 2 counts to lift yourself and the ball and 2 counts to slowly lower down to the ground.

129

BALANCING ON THE BALL
Learn how to manage your body on this unstable surface

Before you start to use the ball to hold you up or do abdominal work, I encourage you to practice getting used to the ball. If you are an intermediate or advanced exerciser, this might be easy. But it might not be easy if you have never tried working with a ball or have never tried stability training. Some people have only ever used machines. I have trained many people who have worked out for years before working with me and could not work with the ball right away. I would

never assume that they had a certain fitness level or capability until I tested it.

Treat each new exercise as if it is a test, and then proceed to learn and implement the exercise step by step. If you assume you can balance yourself on the ball and start one of these exercises before testing it out, you could lose your balance and fall. I have seen it happen. There is no shame when learning something new to be careful with your body.

Ball Chair at Desk

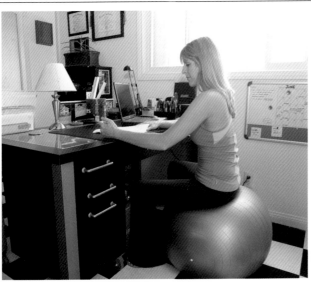

- One good way to get used to the ball is to replace your desk chair with a ball.

- You may not be able to sit on the ball for the entire day, but starting off with an hour or two can help you become comfortable with this new unstable surface.

- There are balls on the market that were created to replace your office desk chair. They can be sized to fit what you need.

- You may experience some fatigue in your spinal muscles as well as your abs after sitting upright with your core engaged all day.

Get Used to the Ball

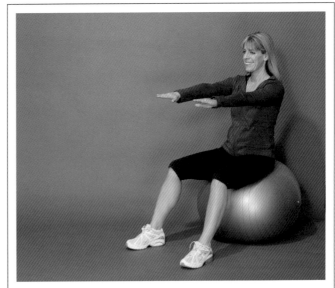

- Before you do crunches on the ball, you need to be able to feel comfortable getting on and off the ball safely.

- Start by sitting upright on the ball in an area that has open space with no sharp objects.

- Sit in the center of the ball and make sure you are comfortable there before moving on.

- You may want to do this on a mat or carpet in case you slide off so you have something soft to land on.

Your exercise program should not cause you injury, but I see it happen all the time. Work smarter first to create a strong foundation of strength and skill, and then work harder to keep getting results.

Walk Yourself Forward

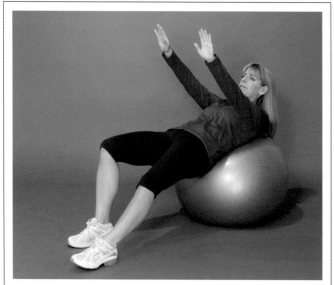

- Once you feel comfortable sitting on the ball, start to walk your legs out in front of you.

- Lower your upper body down to place it on the ball; your abs will work to lower you.

- Take each step slowly and keep yourself centered on the ball.

- This exercise may be difficult enough as it is and can be done over and over as an exercise.

End Position

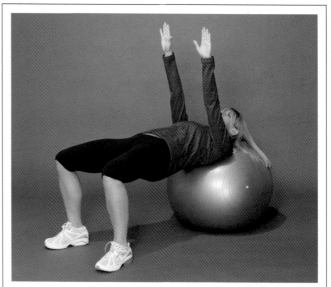

- Walk yourself forward and lower your upper body down until you are lying with your back on the ball.

- If you feel discomfort in your neck, use one hand to support your head. Be careful not to throw off your balance when doing so.

- You can lower down as far as you are comfortable, but you ultimately want to rest your neck on the ball.

- Your lower body will work to help hold you up, so don't be surprised if you feel your legs in this exercise.

CRUNCHES ON THE BALL
Using a ball with a crunch creates more motion

I love using the ball for crunches for three very important reasons.

First, it makes regular crunches seem more exciting after you have been doing them for a while.

Second, your body works not only to lift you but to stabilize you, so more muscle is involved. When you are lying on the ground, your body does not have to do anything, because you are not resisting anything. On the ball, you have to balance the entire time, so the exercise engages more active tissue than on the ground.

Third, and most important to me, is that the ball acts as a fulcrum.

A fulcrum is the point or support on which a lever pivots. In this case the lever is the body weight that you move when you crunch. Why is this important? Do a half crunch upper on the floor and test your active range of motion. Now, roll up a

Beginner Position

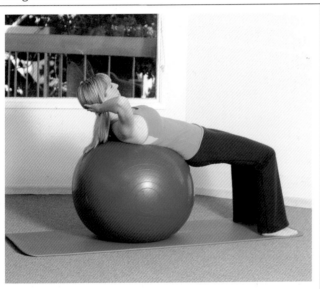

- Your starting position on the ball will determine the exercise's difficulty.

- Keep your feet wide to create a wider base of support. Make sure your feet are flat on the ground and secure. Never do ball work on a slippery floor.

- How much of your upper body is off the ball determines the amount of resistance.

- Start small with only your head and shoulders off the ball.

Intermediate/Advanced Position

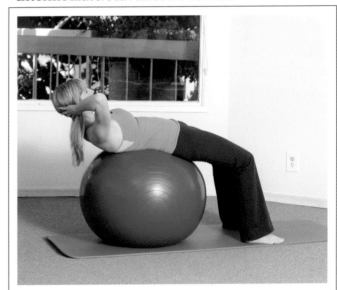

- When you are comfortable and strong enough, walk yourself backward so that more of your upper body hangs over the ball.

- Make sure that at every position you can securely anchor your feet on the ground.

- If you want to make it even harder, extend your arms together over your head to create a longer lever.

- Adjust your resistance and position on the ball so that you can execute the exercise and have enough resistance to make it count.

towel or put a pillow underneath your lower back and do a half crunch upper again. In most cases your active range of motion increases, because in this case the pillow or towel is the fulcrum.

Your lower back has a curvature that does not naturally touch the ground when you're on your back. When you do a crunch, your lower back has to change the curve so your body pushes down against the floor to allow you to pivot at that point and lift yourself up. Adding a ball or towel decreases the distance for the back to move in order for your spine to start flexing. Basically, your abs start working sooner when the back has less distance to move before you pivot. While this may be more science than you need, understanding this concept can help you create other exercises that can increase the amount of effort your abs put into them.

Ball Crunch

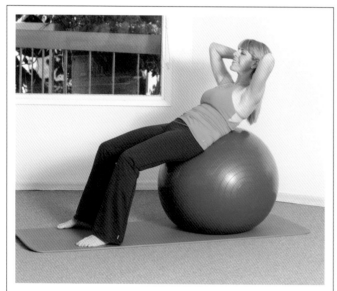

- Find a position on the ball that is comfortable to start.

- Because the ball as a fulcrum creates more spinal extension as well as flexion, you can allow your upper body to gently drape over the back of the ball.

- Initiate the movement from your ribs, which will be even harder in this position due to the increase in resistance.

- Crunch on the ball by pressing down into the ball with your lower back. Do not move the ball when you move.

Ball Crunch with Rotation

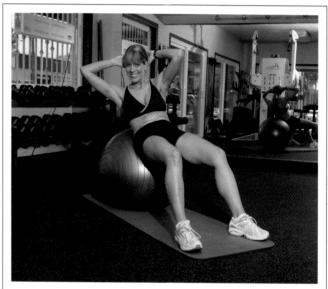

- Use the same form as the ball crunch to start. Decide how much of your body weight you want off the ball.

- Visualize the left half of your abs from your rib cage pulling you up and over toward your right leg.

- Pull yourself up as high as you can go without moving the ball. Use 2 counts and inhale as you pull up.

- Lower down slowly and repeat to the left side using your right ribs to start.

HALF BALL PASS UPPER

Using the ball to focus on can create more movement and use more muscles

I love to create new exercises. Once you know which muscles you want to work, you have so many possibilities for how to move them. Because the abs connect from the rib cage to the pelvis, I like to use each part separately as well as together. You have many options!

This exercise series uses the ball as a prop, which can increase your range of motion or effort level. You can also use a pillow or something of similar size if and when you do not have a ball. I like to create exercises that you can do anywhere and that enable you to use anything to help you. Not many people carry a stability ball with them, so learn this motion and try it with different props such as a pillow, rolled

Start Position

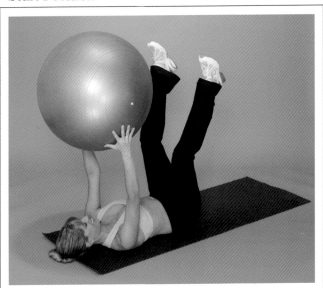

- In this exercise you move only your upper body.

- Start with your legs in the air, with your knees as straight as you can comfortably hold them, and hold the ball in your hands above you.

- You will pass the ball to your legs, but still initiate this move with your ribs.

- Remember that even though you use your arms and legs, the ab work needs to start with the ab muscles.

Pass to Legs

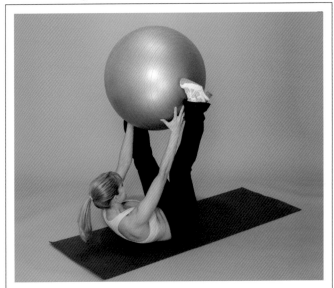

- Pull your upper body to your legs and place the ball in between your legs.

- Use 2 counts and exhale as you lift up to place the ball in between your legs.

- Grab the ball with your legs and hold it there as you lower your upper body to the ground.

- This exercise works the inside of your thighs plus your hips and legs as you hold your lower body up in the air.

up towel or even a stuffed animal! When it comes to creating and executing your ab routine, choose exercises at an appropriate level for your current ability, but try enough variation to choose the ones you like to do best.

If you are a beginner exerciser, you might say you don't like any ab exercises because they are hard work! But once you do them often enough and start to see the results, your relationship to the intensity of the exercises will change, because you will see what they can do for you. When I say you should choose the exercises you like best, use your own criteria but make sure they are challenging enough. Remember: If your body can do it easily, there is no reason for the body to change.

I recommend using an air-filled ball to start these exercises. You can always progress to a weighted ball later if it is appropriate. I would only encourage a weighted ball up to 5 pounds to start.

End Position

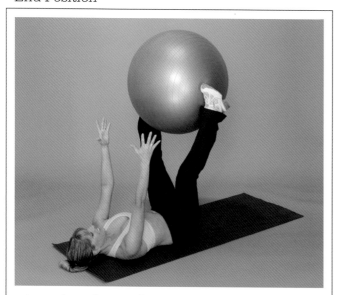

- Lower down after you place the ball in between your legs. There will be nothing in your hands.

- Passing the ball to your legs counts as 1 rep. You will repeat this, but next time your hands will get the ball back from your legs.

- For every other rep, you will pass the ball to the legs or pass the ball back to your hands from your legs.

- This variation keeps this exercise interesting, increases your coordination, and makes the exercise a little harder and maybe even more fun!

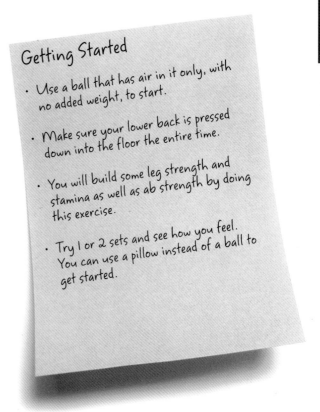

Getting Started

- Use a ball that has air in it only, with no added weight, to start.

- Make sure your lower back is pressed down into the floor the entire time.

- You will build some leg strength and stamina as well as ab strength by doing this exercise.

- Try 1 or 2 sets and see how you feel. You can use a pillow instead of a ball to get started.

HALF BALL PASS LOWER

Use the ball to do additional exercises that work the lower half of your abs

Let's debunk another myth.

You have seen all the illustrations of your ab and core muscles, and I have explained the attachment points of your rib cage and pelvis. The term that gets thrown around that is not 100 percent accurate is "upper and lower abs." Notice, I refer to the lower half or upper half of your abs, but I never section them off from each other by calling them upper abs and lower abs.

People divide the abs into two separate areas based on where they feel an exercise. As you have learned, you can move each side of your body by itself or use both parts at the same time. When I lift my upper body, because my body

Start Position

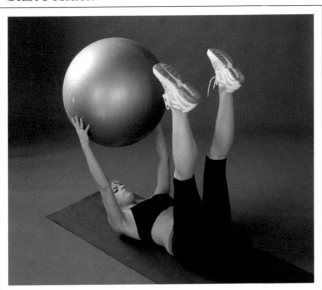

- As in the last exercise, start with your legs in the air and the ball in your hands.

- Your arms should be extended with your hands holding the ball over your head or slightly behind you if you have long legs.

- In this exercise your upper body will stay on the ground and only your lower body will move.

- Try to keep your arms still and do not move them back and forth toward your legs unless you have to in order to execute the exercise.

Mid-Range Position

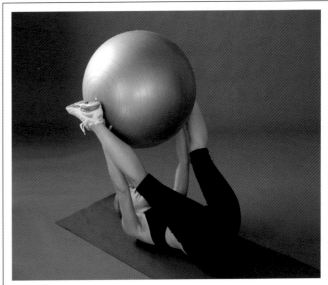

- Draw your lower body closer to your upper body by pulling from your pelvis to your rib cage.

- Use your legs to grab the ball from your hands.

- You need to open your legs wider to fit around the ball and then squeeze.

- You can use a pillow if a ball is too big to start with.

weight force is being moved by the fibers that are closest to my ribs, I feel it in the "upper" part of my abs. That does not mean that my lower half is not working. We have body sensations of difficulty in the muscles that move the force. In this example, the force is the weight of my upper body. Since the abs are long and stabilize the entire body, I will not necessarily feel the fibers closer to my pelvis, but they are working.

I like this exercise because it forces neurological control over your body in a different way. Most of us are familiar with moving the top half of our bodies. This exercise is about moving and isolating the lower half with your abs, which is usually a new or underdeveloped motor pattern. Part of working a set of muscles to increase the strength involves using those muscles in many different patterns to continually progress. I also like it for people who have neck issues or tend to strain their necks in ab exercises.

End Position

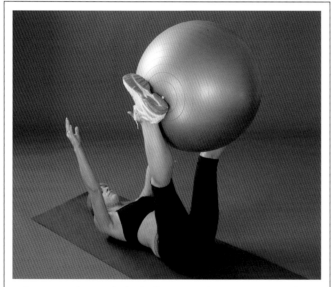

- Bring your legs with the ball or pillow between them back to the start position.

- Do not allow your legs to be so far away from you that your lower back lifts off the ground. Control your legs to return to the start position.

- For the next rep, pass the ball back to your hands and then return the legs without the ball to the start position.

- Pass the ball back and forth by moving only your lower body and concentrating on the lower part of your abs.

Moving Your Lower Body

- Because your lower body weighs more than your upper body, this will be a more challenging exercise.

- Make sure you do this exercise slowly and with control at all times.

- Keep your lower back on the ground when you return to the start position.

- If you cannot control your legs and keep your lower back on the ground, this exercise is too hard for you right now.

JJ'S BALL PASS

Here's an advanced exercise that uses both your upper and lower body in a fun way!

I encourage you to practice the upper and lower half ball passes in this chapter before attempting this advanced exercise. My ball pass is actually a combination of those two exercises. Most intermediate and advanced exercisers have found benefit with this exercise, and I love when I can introduce it to someone new.

This ball pass works your entire core and improves your coordination, leg stamina, and strength. Because you cannot use your hands behind your head, I encourage everyone to try it, but do not force yourself to continue if you start to feel discomfort in your neck. Remember that your head weighs approximately 12 pounds, so your neck muscles will work,

Start Position

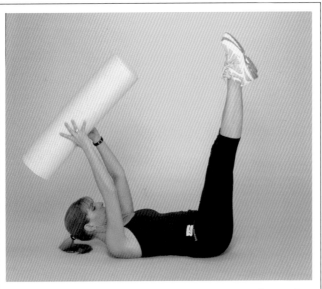

- Grab the ball or pillow with your hands.

- Start with the legs in the air and your lower back pressed down into the floor or mat.

- You are going to be passing the ball or pillow back and forth from your upper to lower body and reverse.

- Maintain control in all your movements and do not throw your body; pull your body slowly and consciously.

Pass to the Legs

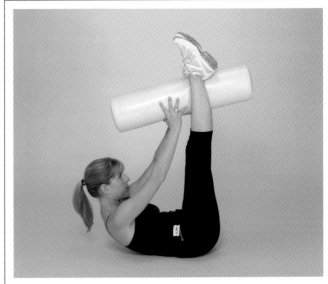

- Pull both sides of your body into the center with your abs.

- Pass the ball or pillow from your hands to your legs; grab the ball or pillow with your legs.

- Squeeze and hold the ball or pillow with your legs as you return to the start position.

- Control your legs so that you do not extend too far away and cannot keep your lower back on the ground.

but you should not experience sharp, shooting pain or head-aches as a result.

Once you have mastered the upper and lower ball passes, this exercise will serve as a natural progression. Using a prop, such as the ball or a pillow, can actually increase your motion, because you concentrate on a bigger arc of motion than without the prop. You use more muscles and need increased brain activity to coordinate the movements and activate the right muscles.

Back to Neutral

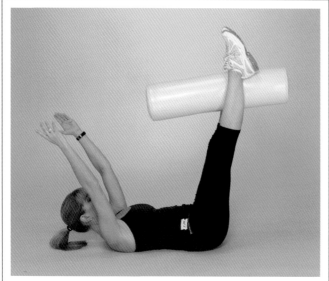

- Return to the start position; now your legs are holding the ball or pillow.

- Keep your arms up and over your head to create more resistance for your upper body.

- Make sure to keep exhal-ing. If you keep your mouth open, you will breathe naturally. Do not hold your breath.

- Take 2 counts in each direction or more. Slower is better.

Pass to Hands

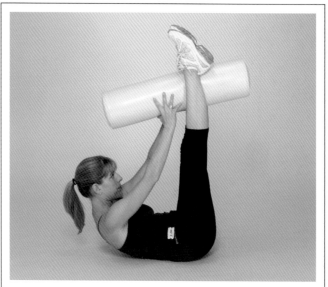

- Pull both sides of your body back into the middle.

- Grab the ball or pillow from your legs with your hands.

- Make sure you exhale and keep your lower back on the floor.

- Use 2 counts in each direc-tion and return to the start position. Repeat passing the ball or pillow back and forth.

139

WHO, WHAT & WHY?

How Pilates started, why, and how it can benefit you

Joseph Pilates was a German-born gymnast. In 1912 he worked as a self-defense instructor for detectives at Scotland Yard. During World War I he started rigging springs to hospital beds to help bed-ridden patients exercise with resistance. The amazing aspect about Pilates' method was that the patients who he trained were among the largest group of survivors during an influenza epidemic, which confirmed his belief that mental health and physical health are connected.

Joseph Pilates created the Pilates Principles for exercising the whole body, which include proper alignment, centering, control, concentration, precision, breathing, and flowing movement. He originally called it Contrology because of the emphasis on the idea that the mind controls the body. The Pilates method teaches awareness of breath and body alignment, with emphasis on the spine as well as on working and strengthening all the core muscles.

Open Leg Balance, Start

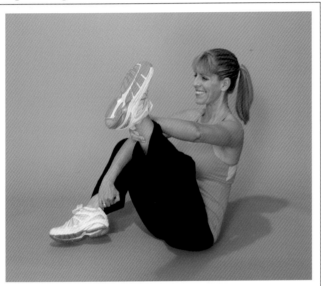

- This is an intermediate to advanced mat exercise, so take your time and use controlled movements.

- Sit up tall on a mat and bring your feet toward your body, knees open, and feet together in a V shape.

- Grab your ankles from the inside of you legs. Keep your chest up and shoulders back.

- Keep pulling your spine up toward the ceiling and think of being tall. Pull in your abs and imagine lifting them up.

Open Leg Balance, Finish

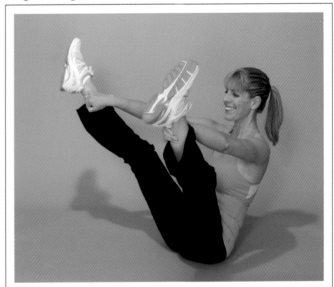

- With control, extend your left leg in the air first and straighten it.

- Find your balance before extending the right leg. Make sure you are not on your tailbone but slightly forward.

- Hold this position while thinking of pulling your abs in and up for a count of 5 or 10.

- Gently release one leg at a time to end the exercise or to rest between reps.

Pilates wrote two books about his method: *Return to Life Through Contrology* in 1928 and *Your Health: A Corrective System of Exercising That Revolutionizes the Entire Field of Physical Education* in 1934. Pilates passed away in 1967 at the age of eighty-seven, but his students became teachers and taught others to become teachers to keep this method alive. In the late 1980s, the media created some buzz about the Pilates method, and we have been riding the wave ever since.

One of my favorite aspects about Pilates is the concentration and attention required to perform the exercises. I use these principles with all the exercises I create and with all the clients I train. Pilates is mostly core training, so when you take a class, you can expect to improve your strength, stamina, and awareness of your core. Pilates is a great addition to any program and is popular with dancers because of the similar moves.

Open Leg Rocker, Start

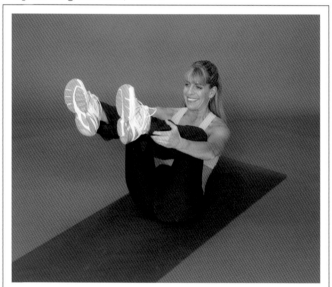

- This is a rolling exercise. Follow the directions for open leg balance; sit up tall, activate your abs, and gently grab one leg or ankle at a time.

- As you find your balance, keep pulling your abs in and up and hold your legs shoulder width apart.

- You do not need to have straight legs; you can keep a slight bend in your knees.

- Take a deep inhalation and draw in your abs to prepare to roll.

Open Leg Rocker, Finish

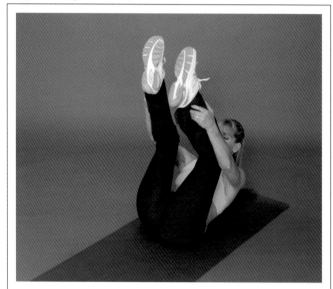

- Exhale and roll back. Concentrate on the contact between your lower back and the floor as you roll back onto your shoulders, keeping your body in a C the entire time.

- Do not throw yourself backward. Use your abs to maintain control of your body.

- Keep your arms and legs in the same position the whole time as you rock up and down.

- Use your breathing and abs to initiate returning to the start position.

MAT VS. REFORMER
Pilates can be done on a machine or on a mat

I do not know any other exercise method that has as many exercises with formal names as Pilates. Do not use the name of the exercise as a guide to what or how to do the exercise. As you will see later in this chapter, I name exercises by what action they use in the body, and Pilates has a new name for each version.

What is the difference between mat and Reformer Pilates? Well, to start out, the Reformer is a machine that offers many different levers and springs to help add resistance to the movements and create movements you could not do on a mat. That does not mean it is better, it just means it is different. The advantage of mat Pilates is that it can be done virtually anywhere, and you really do not even need a mat. Carpet or a soft surface will work just fine.

I use mat exercises with my clients, because I feel it is a good way to get to know your body. Since you use your body

Leg Circles on Mat, Start

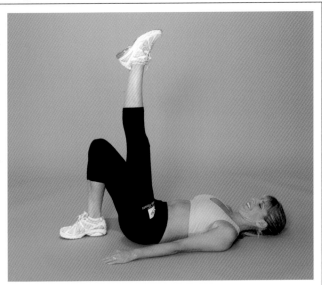

- Lie on the floor on your back with one leg in the air and the other extended.

- Pull in your abs and imagine them stabilizing the ribs and pelvis together.

- Straighten the leg in the air as much as possible but don't lift the hips off the ground to do it. A slight bend in the knee is fine.

- If extending the leg on the ground causes discomfort, bend your knee and put a flat foot on the ground.

Mat Leg Circles Mid-Range

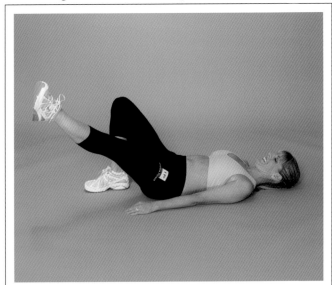

- You will draw a circle with your raised leg in clockwise and counterclockwise directions.

- With your abs pulled in and lower back on the floor, start by drawing a small clockwise circle.

- If you can keep your hips

stabilized and not have them moving all around when you do this, try making a bigger circle, taking 2 to 3 counts to do it.

- Complete 10 circles and then reverse to counterclockwise and repeat. Switch legs and do the sequence on the other leg.

weight as your resistance, learning how to handle and control it is good training to prepare for harder exercises later in your exercise program. One of the biggest mistakes people make in their progression is skipping the smaller steps that can truly accelerate body control and awareness. You have more available muscle and better neurological connection for the harder stuff when you start with the basics of body weight resistance and control.

A Reformer can be fun and interesting. Pilates studios and other venues offer classes and private sessions, and there are home units, which aren't as big or fancy as those in a studio, that can be a great tool for home exercise. I encourage you to try both mat and Reformer Pilates to see what works best for you by taking a class or having a private session to learn how to properly and safely use the Reformer and all of its parts and gadgets.

Reformer Leg Circles, Start

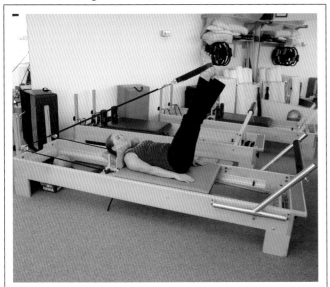

- On a Reformer you have a few options as to how much resistance you want to use for each exercise.

- Have someone who understands the Reformer show you how to adjust the springs and choose an easy to moderate resistance to start.

- Place the foot of the leg you'll be working through the loop on the Reformer; follow the same body form for stabilizing as you would on the ground.

Reformer Leg Circles Mid-Range

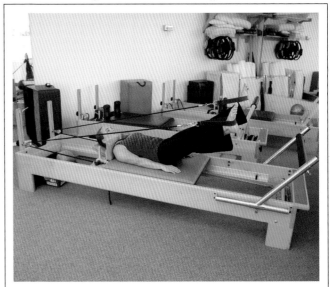

- Gravity and your leg weight are the resistance in mat Pilates. On the Reformer, the resistance comes from the springs.

- Keep your circles consistent; increase the size as long as you can maintain full control over your pelvis.

- In Pilates work you may be guided to do only a few reps on each leg, but it all depends on your goal.

BEGINNER MOVES

The roll up and 100s are basic beginner moves that increase balance and flexibility

I use these two exercises myself and with clients, because even though they are beginner moves, they can be hard for any exerciser who has never moved like a gymnast or dancer. People usually gravitate toward exercises that feel good because they are good at them. Adding new kinds of movements can increase your active range of motion for all your

joints as well as increase your flexibility.

You can do the roll up as a warm-up for your spine and abs, and you can do it on the Reformer as well as on the floor. To make the roll up harder, take more time to lower yourself down and roll back up. Start with aiming to lower yourself for 4 to 6 seconds and roll up for 4 to 6 counts. Once you can do

Roll Up, Start

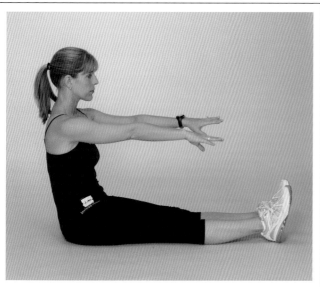

- Sit on the floor with your legs extended in front of you.

- Sit upright as tall as you can and draw your abs in and up.

- Extend your arms in front of you.

- In this exercise, you are going to roll down slowly. Inhale before you start and exhale as you start to move.

Roll Up, Finish

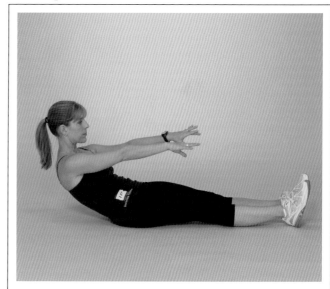

- Visualize your spine and each vertebra. Tuck your pelvis and try to lower your tailbone to the floor first.

- After you place your tailbone on the ground, gently place each vertebra, one at a time, down on the ground as well.

- Once you've rolled all the way down, inhale again and start to lift yourself back up, beginning with your head and neck. Return to a seated position as slowly as you lowered yourself down.

that well, increase the time it takes to roll down or roll up to 8 or 10 seconds and feel the increase of intensity on your abs.

The 100s exercise is harder because it is an isometric exercise, so you have to squeeze your abs for over a minute. Make sure you are comfortable with lifting your upper body off the ground with no neck support. Tuck your head and chin as much as you can to alleviate unnecessary force on your neck. Try using your abs to lift your upper body as high off the ground as you can—this can also help take pressure off your neck. When deciding where to hold your legs, remember that the closer your legs are to you, the easier on your back it will be. If the angle is too much for you, pull your legs closer to the ceiling so they are straighter up and down, or hold them in tabletop like in the start position.

You can slightly adjust any exercise to make it more comfortable and customize it to your body. But if you need to make too many changes, you might try a different exercise altogether.

100s, Start

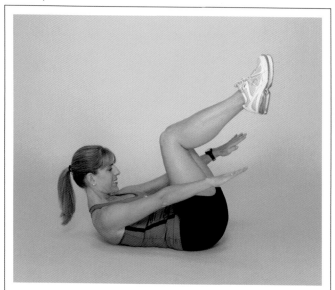

- This is an isometric exercise for the abs; you add resistance with your legs and arms.

- Lie on your back with your knees in tabletop position.

- Lift your arms off the ground and extend them forward; lift your head and chest in an isometric crunch, holding your upper body up off the floor.

- Keep your lower back on the ground and continue to breathe throughout the exercise.

100s, Finish

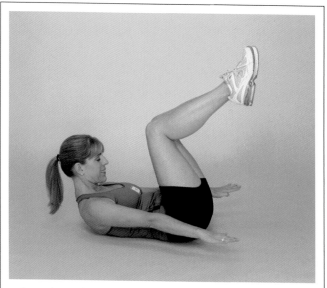

- Extend your legs at a 45-degree angle if you can, or bring them closer if that's easier; you need to be able to hold them throughout the exercise.

- Begin to "flap" your extended arms in a small, staccato motion, or up and down, very quickly and

count each "flap."

- The name of the exercise is 100s, so continue to count each "flap" until you reach 100.

- Exhale and count aloud to be sure you're breathing and keeping track of where you are in the exercise.

145

SINGLE LEG PULL

You use your leg as resistance on your abs in this popular Pilates mat exercise

I learned a series of ab exercises in a mat class years ago that I still love to use today for both myself and in building a program for others. In this ab series, there are four different positions for the same basic exercise, and this is the starting position. This exercise also requires that you use your arms to hold your legs, but you can use one hand behind your head to help with neck support if needed.

There are two things to concentrate on with this exercise. First, keep your abs tight and contracted the whole time—think shortening of the ab muscles. Second, you want to think about lengthening your leg as you switch from side to side. Since you bring your knee in as a rest for one leg while

Single Leg Pull, Start

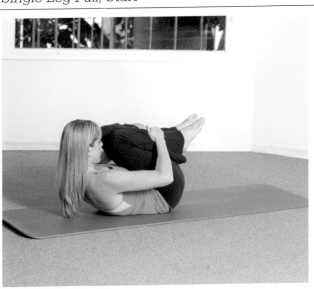

- Grab both knees with your arms and lift your upper body off the ground with your abs at your rib cage.

- Make sure your lower back is pressed into the ground and you are as tucked as you can be.

- Even though you are moving your arms and legs, remember to focus on your abs holding you together and pulling both sides of your body into the middle.

- Inhale before you start and exhale through the mouth each time your switch legs.

Single Leg Pull, Finish

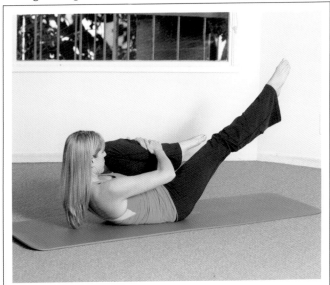

- Extend one leg at a 45-degree angle; grab the other knee with both hands.

- Hold this position with your lower back pressed into the floor for 2 counts and then switch legs.

- As you keep switching legs, remember to hold yourself tightly in the center by using your abs.

- Exhale each time you change legs and aim to do this exercise for at least 60 seconds or 20 to 25 reps on each side.

146

the other is extended, think long and lengthen the leg that is extended.

This exercise is an isometric exercise, because the focus is on keeping the length of your abs the same, while you use your legs as resistance. You will feel work happening in the legs as well as in the abs and even in the arms, because they are helping to lift your upper body.

Protect Your Neck

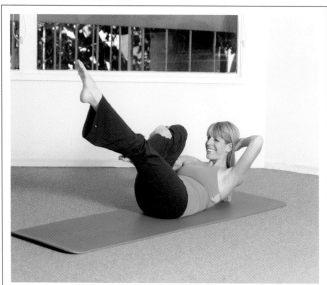

- Test the exercise out first as explained above and see how your body feels.

- Hopefully you feel most of the work in your abs and some in your legs.

- If you feel strain or too much pressure on your neck, use one hand behind your head and one hand for your legs.

- Apply just enough effort to relieve your neck but do not clasp your head or pull on your neck.

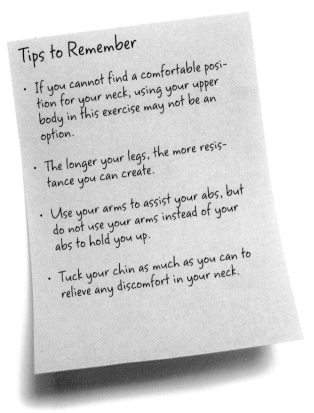

Tips to Remember

- If you cannot find a comfortable position for your neck, using your upper body in this exercise may not be an option.

- The longer your legs, the more resistance you can create.

- Use your arms to assist your abs, but do not use your arms instead of your abs to hold you up.

- Tuck your chin as much as you can to relieve any discomfort in your neck.

DOUBLE LEG STRETCH

Using your upper and lower body as resistance is the most advanced type of exercise

The single leg pull is the first in a series of exercises that I use because it is the easiest version. The double leg stretch is a more advanced version and provides more resistance to your core. This exercise demands both strength and endurance from the abdominals to resist the weight of your entire upper body and lower body at the same time. You can always

modify it by leaving your head down or adjusting the height of your legs. It is helpful to focus on staying very narrow in this exercise. Hold your legs tightly together as they extend away from you, and keep them tight as you pull them back in.

Take notes about the exercises you are doing to track what is working and what is too hard or causes a strange pull or

Double Leg Stretch, Start

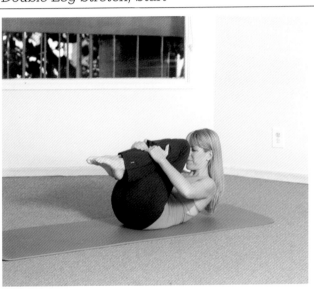

- Lie on your back with your legs in tabletop position, parallel to the floor.

- Pull in your abs and lift your upper body off the ground using your ab muscles.

- Grab your legs on the outside below the knees with your hands and squeeze yourself into a ball.

- Be sure your lower back is in contact with the floor.

Double Leg Stretch, Finish

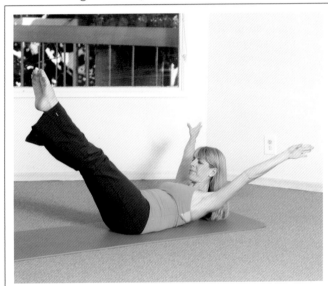

- Reach your arms over your head and stretch your legs out straight.

- Extend and reach as far as possible while keeping your abs pulled in and your lower back on the mat.

- Bring your arms out to your sides, bring in your legs, and grasp your shins to bring your body back to the start position.

- You might need to adjust the height of your arms and legs as you reach. The lower they are, the more difficult it is.

soreness. If you feel your muscles a day or two later, that is a good sign that you are working intensely enough to build some muscle and strength. However, if you continue to feel pain, you may not be doing the exercise properly. Tracking your exercises will also let you know when it is time to progress to the next level, and this exercise is definitely an advanced level.

If you are a beginner, get the single leg pull under your belt before adding this one to your routine. If you are an intermediate or advanced exerciser, try it now and see how well you do. However I cannot emphasize enough the importance of maintaining good form. Throwing your body around can lead to injury, but, more important, your muscles will not benefit from the exercise if you do not use good form. Aim to be efficient so you can feel confident that the time you spend exercising makes a difference.

Protect Your Neck

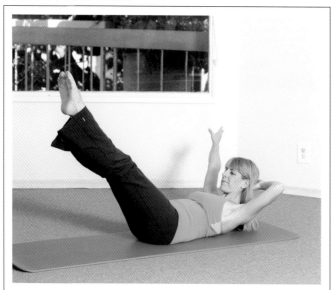

- Use the same form but place one hand behind your head to support your neck.

- You may want to switch hands after every 5 reps to keep your arms from fatiguing.

- Because of the intensity of this exercise, you may try doing the bottom half only and leaving your upper body and head on the ground or a pillow.

- See what works for you, but remember this is an advanced exercise, so work your way up to it.

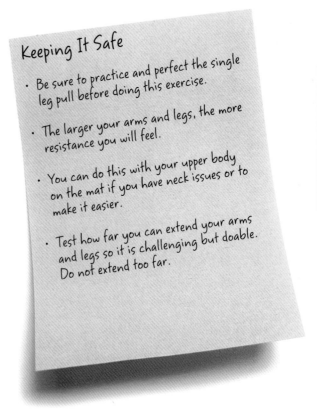

Keeping It Safe

- Be sure to practice and perfect the single leg pull before doing this exercise.

- The larger your arms and legs, the more resistance you will feel.

- You can do this with your upper body on the mat if you have neck issues or to make it easier.

- Test how far you can extend your arms and legs so it is challenging but doable. Do not extend too far.

149

SINGLE STRAIGHT LEG STRETCH

Increase the intensity of the single leg pull on your core by doing this advanced version

Once the single leg pull becomes too easy, graduate to the single straight leg stretch. I do not generally try to focus on a stretch, so don't let the title of this exercise deceive you. It's actually the straight leg version of the single leg pull. The form will be the same, except instead of pulling your knees in to your chest, you will pull in straight legs.

In Pilates, they want you to pull in your leg as far as you can to stretch—I do not. I focus and promote active stretching, which is where your body moves you. A passive stretch is when an outside force other than the muscles in question pushes or pulls you into a range of motion you cannot do by yourself. In this case your arms pull your leg closer to you. It

Start Position

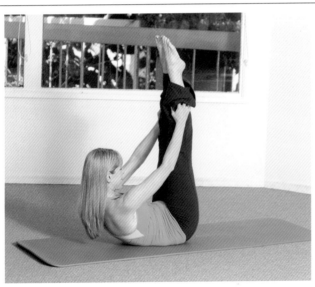

- Lie on the ground with your back on the mat and legs extended toward the ceiling.

- Pull in your abs, tuck your chin, and lift your upper body up off the mat. The tips of your shoulder blades should remain on the mat.

- You will maintain this position throughout the exercise. Use your abs to help pull you up and keep you up.

- Grab your left leg above the knee with both hands.

Left Leg

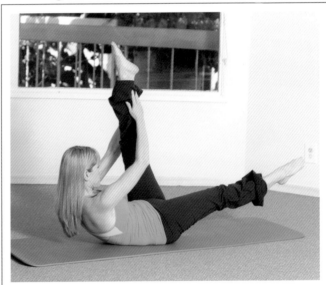

- Extend the right leg out and down at a 45-degree angle.

- Keep your upper body as high as you can while you switch legs. Take 2 counts for each leg.

- Gently pull your right leg toward you. Pulse the leg toward you twice and exhale.

- Switch legs quickly, keeping your upper body high off the mat.

is a passive stretch. Apply some force to pulling your leg in toward your center, but do not pull too hard. Concentrate on the abs more than the leg to make sure you are getting the most out of this for your core.

To create a series of these core exercises, you could start with a set of single leg pulls and then go straight into the single straight leg stretch.

Right Leg

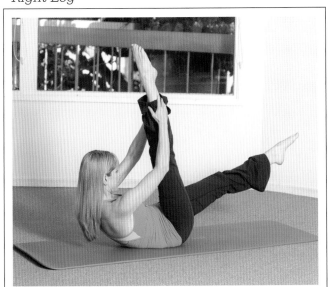

- Grab your right leg and pull it toward you as you lower the left leg out and down.

- If you have long legs and this is very difficult, bend your leg to lessen the resistance.

- Pull the leg in for 2 counts and make sure to continue breathing.

- Switch quickly again and repeat this 10 to 20 times to start before deciding how many you should be doing.

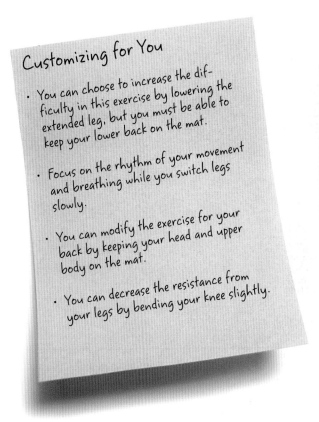

Customizing for You

- You can choose to increase the difficulty in this exercise by lowering the extended leg, but you must be able to keep your lower back on the mat.

- Focus on the rhythm of your movement and breathing while you switch legs slowly.

- You can modify the exercise for your back by keeping your head and upper body on the mat.

- You can decrease the resistance from your legs by bending your knee slightly.

PILATES

WHY USE MACHINES?

There are reasons for and against using machines to enhance your exercise

When people think of working out, the majority probably visualize exercising in a gym. Most gyms have machines and equipment for nearly all parts of the body, ranging from simple and small to large and complex. Some people want to know which is better, machines or free weights. And the answer is neither and both. Let's look at the reasons why you would want to use a machine in the gym and why you would choose not to.

On a simple level, if you are a beginner, you may need some guidance as to what to do. Some machines may provide instructions that would help you decide if you need what it offers, and it may even guide you on how to use it. Machines

Machine Is Too Big

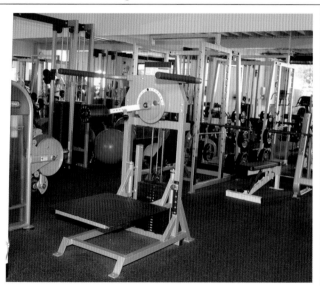

- There are several lines of gym equipment built for sport-specific training and bodies.

- Some of these machines are built for very large men.

- A small-framed female cannot fit on the same machine

- and might find the range of motion uncomfortable.

- Some machines are adjustable, so you may be able to adapt them to your body size. Some are not adjustable; do not force an exercise on a piece of equipment that you can feel is too large for you.

Machines for Every Body

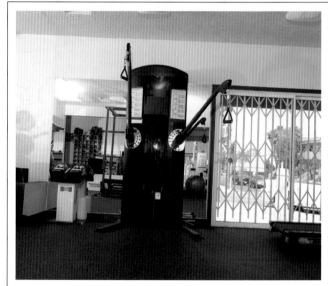

- There are a few lines of equipment for both home and gym that have arms that swivel, rotate, and adjust for almost any motion you want to create.

- Although these pieces may be large, they adjust for everyone. To use them, you need to know the kind

- of motion or exercise you want to create.

- Once you learn the exercises and motions you want to create, you might only need this one piece of equipment, as it is so versatile.

provide stability in certain situations and also can administer low to high levels of resistance if appropriate. Machines can apply resistance in places and ways that you cannot achieve in gravity. All of these are good reasons to use machines in your exercise program.

Why might you not want to use a machine? If there are no instructions, it may be more detrimental than beneficial if you get injured using a piece of equipment incorrectly or with bad form. Machines have permanent axis and range of motion capabilities. If you do not fit the same range or

motion or size of the machine, you could put wear and tear on your joints. Machines stabilize your body weight for you a lot of the time, so you are not required to use your stabilizers. This will not necessary hurt you, but learning how to stabilize your own body weight while doing an exercise can increase your core strength and balance.

The bottom line is to be smart and learn about the machines, what they do, and why you may or may not want to use them.

Cable Cross

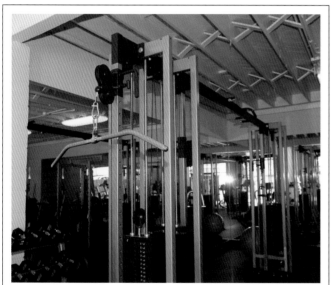

- Cables are a great way to redirect resistance to create exercises that are not gravity based.

- You can do them standing up, seated, bent over, lying down, from the side, and more.

- All the different attach- ments and handles give you a variety of ways to use the machine to create exercises that are right for you.

- Because of the versatility, you won't find instructions on a cable machine. Ask for help and/or a demonstration before performing the exercises.

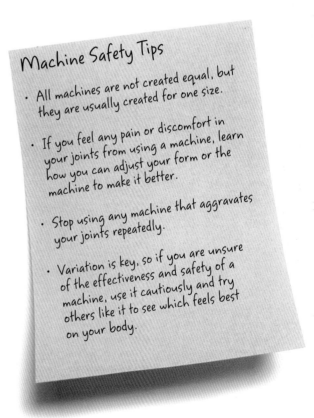

Machine Safety Tips

- All machines are not created equal, but they are usually created for one size.

- If you feel any pain or discomfort in your joints from using a machine, learn how you can adjust your form or the machine to make it better.

- Stop using any machine that aggravates your joints repeatedly.

- Variation is key, so if you are unsure of the effectiveness and safety of a machine, use it cautiously and try others like it to see which feels best on your body.

THE GOOD & THE BAD

Exploring the deeper reasons why you may or may not choose to use an exercise machine

Now let's consider the more advanced reasons why you may and may not want to use machines to help you exercise. First, if you are in some way limited in range of motion or have a preexisting condition that affects your balance or strength, then a machine might be appropriate. For example, if you have trouble lying on your back or you have a neck injury that is aggravated when you lie down, using one of the machines that enables you to work your abs while seated could help you continue to exercise. When you do abs on the ground, gravity serves as your resistance. When you stand up or are seated upright, you need a machine or tool to create resistance in a different plane in order for you to work this muscle.

Machines with Neck Support

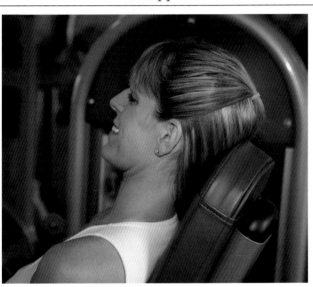

- Machines that support your neck can feel comfortable at first, whether you're doing an ab exercise or working another body part.

- Having neck support might be appropriate if every exercise you attempt hurts your neck.

- If you can hold your neck in certain ab exercises, you may want to continue to strengthen it by not relying on a machine to hold it for you.

- Work on perfect form for ab exercises and you may find that you don't need the extra support.

Using Upright Ab Machines

- If you have severe back problems when you lie on your back, finding an upright substitute would be useful.

- The problem with these machines is that most people do not use good form, because they rely on the machine to support them.

- Regardless of what kind of machine you use, always think of pulling your abs together from your rib cage, pelvis, or both.

- Machines supply the resistance; to be safe and effective, you are responsible for good form.

154

Now let's look at why you may not want to use a machine. If you feel your neck is weak and it always hurts when you do ab exercises, you may consider using a machine that holds your neck for you. This could be a problem for a few reasons. First, if you have an average neck length and can bring your chin to your chest or close to it, you may need to work on your form so that you don't engage your neck. Too many people pull from their neck instead of their ribs and put more pressure on their neck than is needed. Second, your head weighs around 12 pounds. Your neck muscles need to work to hold up you head. If you use a machine to do this for you, you will never increase your neck strength because the machine will always provide a crutch. You disproportionately gain strength by building really strong abs, but you never strengthen the neck muscles.

Create Your Own

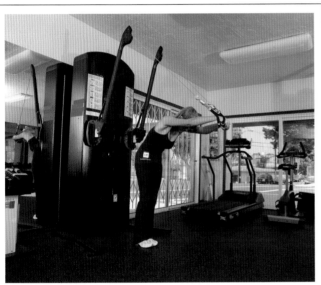

- If you have a fear of discomfort when using your neck, you can create an upright ab exercise. Adjust the arms of the machine over your head. Hold the cable with both hands and do a crunch standing up by moving only from your rib cage.

- Start with a light weight and do 25 to 30 reps. Do not to use your arms, and use the same control and focus you would on the ground.

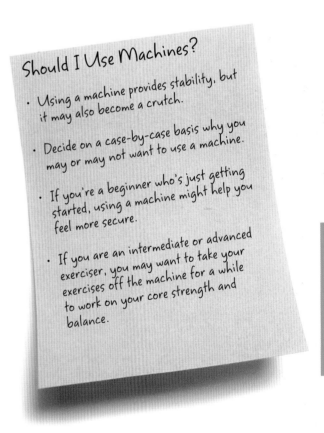

Should I Use Machines?

- Using a machine provides stability, but it may also become a crutch.

- Decide on a case-by-case basis why you may or may not want to use a machine.

- If you're a beginner who's just getting started, using a machine might help you feel more secure.

- If you are an intermediate or advanced exerciser, you may want to take your exercises off the machine for a while to work on your core strength and balance.

MAKE A PLAN

To achieve your fitness and weight-loss goals, you need to make a plan

If I wanted to drive from Los Angeles to Oklahoma City, where I have never been before, and I did not have a GPS, how would I get there? I would need a map. What does this have to do with exercise? If you have a goal for your body that you have never achieved or have not achieved in many years, you need a map—or a plan—to get there.

Start by defining your goals in the most specific and measureable ways possible. "To be healthy" is not a specific enough goal. Ask ten people what healthy means to them and you might get ten different answers. Your goals need to be measurable such as pounds lost, number of stairs you can climb, decreased heart rate, or inches lost. How will you

Beginning with Machines

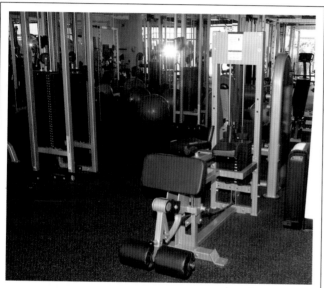

- When you don't know if a machine is right for you, be cautious and work slowly with control.

- Start with a weight you can use for 20 to 25 reps at a slow 4-count rep speed. This means count 2 seconds in one phase of the exercise and 2 seconds in the other.

- Try several sets in a row, up to 3, and check in with your body about what you feel. Make sure you feel it mostly in your muscles, not your joints.

Free Weights

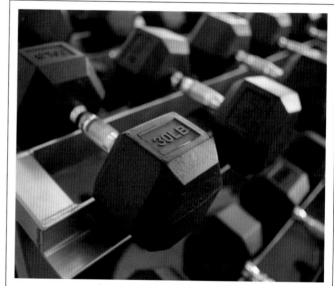

- The next step would be to learn the equivalent exercise with free weights.

- Free weights provide nothing but resistance. You have to stabilize your own body and control the path and range of motion.

- Free weights allow you to

create motions that match your body more personally than a machine, but you have to be prepared to understand and have control over the motions you make.

- If you become advanced at using free weights, you can progress to the next level.

know you when you've achieved a goal if you have no way to measure it?

Next you have to make a plan to get to that goal from where you are now. When it comes to incorporating machines into your program, I can provide a simple progression model that you can use. After you decide on the muscles you want to work in your program, you can choose what exercises to do to work them.

Stability Ball

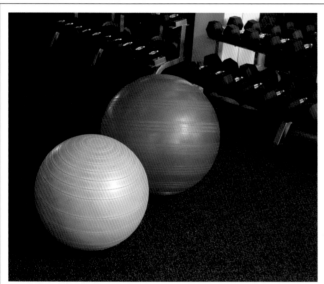

- A ball provides instability, which we covered earlier in Chapter 12.

- Exercises on a ball are considered advanced because you have to stabilize your body as you do the motion and you also have to work extra hard to stabilize on unstable ground.

- You can attempt exercising with a ball or free weights earlier, but use lighter weight or resistance to gain control over the motions first.

- Once you master the ball, you can add more resistance to build more muscle and strength.

Steps of the Plan

- Outline your vision in several different ways to measure your goals and progress.

- Create your map by writing down the first steps you plan to take. You will use the FITT principle later to assist with this in Chapter 18.

- Choose your exercises and machines and chart the weight and sets you start with.

- Make sure to progress to the next level once you feel you can do an exercise with ease and little struggle.

MACHINES

ADDING RESISTANCE

Adding resistance to your exercises can make them harder when appropriate

When is it appropriate to add resistance? When it comes to most muscle groups, I would suggest that the moment you can do your exercises with a great amount of ease and no struggle, it is time to increase or add resistance. Remember that when the body can do an exercise with no problem, there is no reason for the body to change.

Now when it comes to ab work, I am not a fan of adding large amounts of resistance, and here's why: It's your core's job to keep your upper and lower body attached. The core muscles hold, protect, and move your spine forward, backward, and side to side. These muscles are thin, flat, and long and do not have a lot of "bulk" to them naturally because

Cable Weight Stack

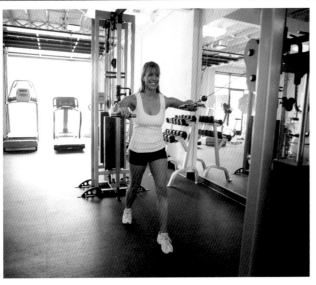

- If you're in a gym, the most common versatile machine is the cable crossover.

- Cables allow you to redirect the way you use resistance that is not dictated by gravity.

- The easiest plate may be 5 or 10 pounds, and that may be enough. The exercise shown here is advanced but different enough to give you an idea of what is possible. I would not add resistance until you have maximized your body weight potential.

Tubing

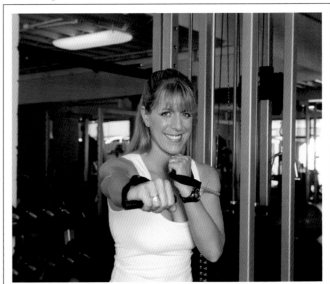

- Tubing is a much safer option; you can add lighter resistance but also add speed or explosion without inertia.

- If you want to work on the speed or intensity of a boxing move or rotation movement, tubing is safer on your joints than free

- weights and machines. Make sure to secure the tubing in a place opposite your motion in the same plane.

- Use all the form and technique you would normally, starting slowly and working up to faster moves.

they were meant to be stabilizers. They are actually the number one group of stabilizers in your body. So we treat them like stabilizers, not like prime movers.

If you look at some of the other muscles in the body, like the pectoralis major (the chest) or quadriceps (the thighs), you'll notice that they are large, fan-shaped muscles with a thicker midsection. These are prime movers; their job is to move the legs or arms and anything we have in our arms. The abs are there to help these muscles do their job by stabilizing the spine and creating a strong foundation from which to produce force. When it comes to adding extra resistance to your abs, I am going to say that it is not necessary in most cases, and you can get plenty of resistance with your body weight alone. However, for those cases that could benefit from added resistance, like bodybuilding or sport-specific goals, here are some options and safe ways to do it.

Resistance and Abs

- Adding resistance to ab work is normally not necessary when you are a beginner or intermediate exerciser.

- If you have a sport-specific goal, are a bodybuilder, or have a specific reason to add resistance to your abs, do it carefully and progress slowly.

- Remember your ab muscles are not the same kind of muscles as your biceps and hamstrings, so they will not be able to "bulk" up to the same proportion as your prime movers.

Your Anatomy

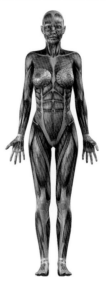

- Just by looking at the body, you can see the difference between the size, shape, and position of all the different muscles.

- The surface muscles and larger muscles are considered prime movers. They are thicker and larger because they have more power.

- The thinner and smaller muscles are stabilizers. They usually have a higher endurance but cannot produce massive amounts of force like the prime movers can.

- Take some time to learn anatomy; it can really enhance your workout!

HOW MUCH & HOW OFTEN

Your existing fitness level will determine how often you may want to use a machine or gadget

As discussed, there are reasons for and against using machines. I have a new client who is 90 years old. In addition to the genetics she inherited to keep her in such great shape, she has exercised over the years to keep herself strong. When she had a goal to lose weight, she started to add cardio to her exercise program until she lost the weight. She adjusted

her food, too, and has kept the weight off. She recently shared with me that she used to have more weight around her middle. She used a machine for her abs that I would have never recommended because I think it's a gimmick. She used it once a day for 3 months. She swears that this machine helped her to lose the weight around her middle,

Ab Wheels or Ball

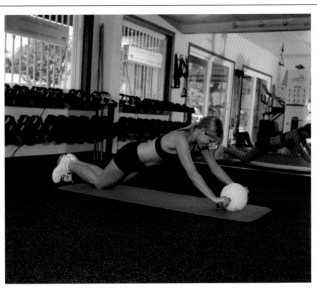

- Because these gadgets are advanced, I would suggest doing 1 set of 10 to 20 reps of rolling the ball forward and backward.

- Start on your knees with your hands on the handles.

- Keep your abs tight and posture stabilized; allow your body to roll forward.

- Use your abs to pull you back to your knees. If this is very hard, aim to do 1 set of 10 to 20 reps every 2 to 3 days. Increase the number of reps when you get stronger.

Cables and Machines

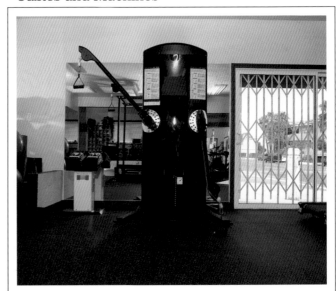

- Depending on what exercise you are doing on the machine and your fitness level, I recommend 2 to 3 sets per week.

- In order to gain control over your body, always start with the basic ab exercises in this book without a machine.

- Try one machine at a time and add 2 to 3 sets per week to your routine. Do the same machine for at least 3 to 4 weeks before moving to a new one.

and it has never come back. Do I believe her? Yes. I believe that she used this machine while she was also doing cardio and changing her diet and that all three components helped her to get great results.

A lot of your experience with exercise will be how you perceive it. My client expected great things to happen, and they did. In her mind the machine did the magic. Personally I believe her powerful decision to take action, her commitment to her body, and a balanced program made it happen.

Should you use a machine to enhance your ab exercises? If it will inspire you to do the exercises and love them, then by all means. Just be sure to use the science you've learned to set realistic expectations. If you are just beginning to exercise, you might need more time to reach your goals than intermediate and advanced exercisers, but remember that the determining factor for your program is your goal.

Multi Hip Machine

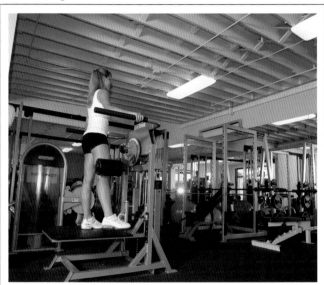

- This versatile machine is not meant for abs directly, but you will need to have strong abs to stabilize your body.

- The hips are also important core stabilizers, and you will need strong abs to do these exercises properly.

- You can get a great ab workout on machines that challenge your balance because your abs help stabilize your spine.

- Do at least 2 to 3 exercises a week that challenge your balance and do 2 to 3 sets of each exercise.

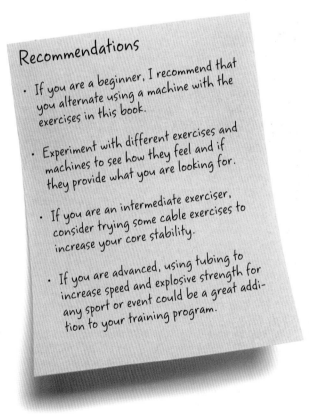

Recommendations

- If you are a beginner, I recommend that you alternate using a machine with the exercises in this book.

- Experiment with different exercises and machines to see how they feel and if they provide what you are looking for.

- If you are an intermediate exerciser, consider trying some cable exercises to increase your core stability.

- If you are advanced, using tubing to increase speed and explosive strength for any sport or event could be a great addition to your training program.

INCREASING METABOLISM

Your nervous system and muscular system make up your resting metabolism. Which should you focus on?

I love talking about metabolism, because it is related to one of the biggest mistakes people—especially women—make with exercise. First let's talk about what metabolism is. Your resting metabolism is the number of calories (energy) your body needs every day just to function. You can find out what your resting metabolism is with a simple equation after you

know your body fat percentage, or you can get it tested on one of several body composition machines. This number is a reflection of two major systems in your body that require energy at rest: the nervous system and muscular system.

The nervous system component is usually just genetics, and you can tell how fast yours is by how you are in life. If you

Fat-Burning Pills = Dangerous

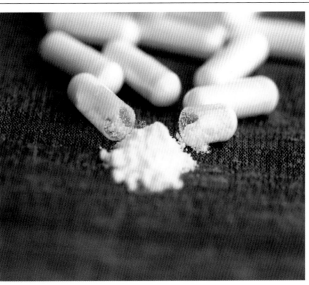

- Most fat-burning pills contain caffeine, or herbs that act like caffeine, to stimulate your nervous system.

- These pills are dangerous and only work short-term. Once you stop taking them, your nervous system returns to normal and you could gain back lost weight.

- Taxing your nervous system can potentially damage your hormones and cause adrenal fatigue. This makes losing weight even harder.

- Caffeine also puts a strain on your nervous system and hormones over time.

Green Tea

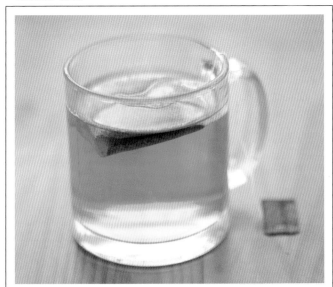

- Green tea has been called one of the best natural fat burners around.

- It contains caffeine but much less than coffee or herbs.

- Green tea is loaded with antioxidants, which can help prevent signs of aging.

- You can find powders that have green tea extract in them and add them to shakes. I take a supplement that has green tea in it. Or you can replace your cup of coffee with a cup of green tea!

are a type A personality and always on the go, talk fast, think fast, and so on, you need a lot of energy to keep up that pace. If you are more like the "surfer dude" who moves, eats, and thinks slowly, your nervous system does not need as much energy as a type A person.

I suggest not trying to change your metabolism through your nervous system, because it is short-term and dangerous. Instead, focus on building muscle to increase your metabolism (see Chapter 8).

Cayenne Pepper

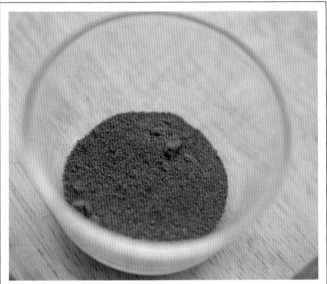

- Ever eat something spicy and start to sweat? Hot spices like cayenne are natural metabolism boosters.

- Your metabolism is only affected when you are consuming these food items, so the effect is temporary, but adding them to your diet can make a difference.

- If you don't like spicy foods, consider taking a supplement that contains cayenne pepper for a natural, caffeine-free boost.

- Try new dishes and get creative so you can enjoy more foods that have a fat-burning effect!

Cinnamon

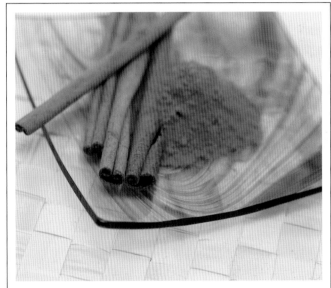

- A sweet way to boost your metabolism is with cinnamon. There are many ways to get cinnamon into your diet.

- You can start the day by adding cinnamon to a shake, oatmeal, or yogurt.

- Cinnamon tea is a great way to get a boost in the afternoon.

- Adding cinnamon to rice pudding, cookies, apple crisp, and other desserts can also help your body digest your food better. You can also take a supplement that contains cinnamon.

163

IT ALL COUNTS!

RESISTANCE TRAINING

Maintaining weight loss is easier when you increase your metabolism by adding resistance training

This is my favorite topic. For over 13 years, I have been helping men and women build muscle and increase their metabolism through resistance training. The greatest obstacle is the image many people have when they think about resistance training. They often visualize a bodybuilder and decide they don't want to be that big. Achieving that kind of body involves much more than just resistance training.

We have over three hundred muscles and over two hundred bones in our bodies. We have so many because we were born to move, not sit. How many of your muscles do you use each day? How many of them do you challenge?

Resistance training involves adding resistance to move-

Biceps Curl

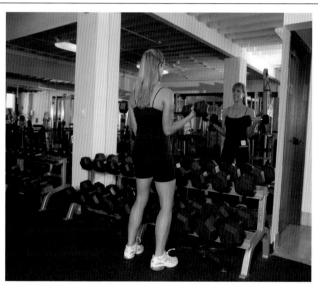

- When you add resistance to a muscle, you want the muscle to fatigue and get bigger and stronger.

- Working the small muscles of the arms can shape and tighten the arms, but it won't make dramatic increases in metabolism.

- Work both sides of your arms and train all sides of your joints to keep them strong and balanced.

- For the average person, I recommend a minimum of 3 sets of three different biceps exercises 1 day a week.

Triceps Press

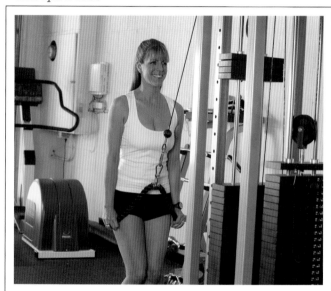

- The triceps are located on the back of the arms; they're the ones that may flap in the wind when you wave.

- The triceps consists of three muscles, while the biceps has two. Keeping the triceps strong also helps with shoulder movement.

- There are many exercises for triceps, but be careful on your shoulder joint.

- I recommend doing 3 sets of three different triceps exercises at least 1 day a week.

ments to stimulate the muscles to build. Your metabolism is like your gas tank. How big is your gas tank? Imagine a Hummer and an Escort—which has the bigger gas tank? The Hummer does, because it is bigger and has more metal, so it needs more energy to make it move. When you add muscle, you increase your body's need for energy. Other benefits of resistance training include increased bone density, strength, and endurance—which can also prevent injury—and a tighter, firmer look that we all love. It does not mean big, bulky muscles.

Another fact to consider is that you lose muscle every year after about the age of 35 if you do not actively put it on. That means that if you weigh 125 at age 25 and do no resistance training until age 35, then even though the scale may still say 125, you have lost approximately 10 pounds of muscle and gained 10 pounds of fat. The scale just tells you your mass number, not how much fat, muscle, or water you have.

Shoulder Fly

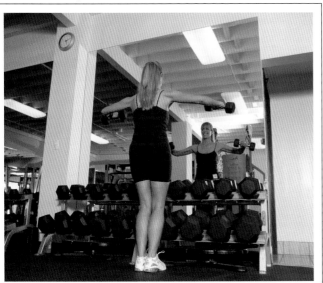

- Your deltoids have three sections: anterior, posterior, and medial. This exercise works mostly the anterior and medial, but the posterior helps to stabilize the shoulder joint while you do it.

- Having shoulder strength is important especially as you

age. Keep your shoulders strong, but be careful how you work them, because the joint is easily injured.

- Do not throw the weight when doing this exercise; pull it very slowly and think of using your shoulders, not your arms, to do it.

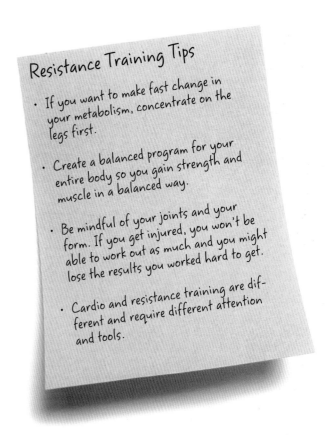

Resistance Training Tips

- If you want to make fast change in your metabolism, concentrate on the legs first.

- Create a balanced program for your entire body so you gain strength and muscle in a balanced way.

- Be mindful of your joints and your form. If you get injured, you won't be able to work out as much and you might lose the results you worked hard to get.

- Cardio and resistance training are different and require different attention and tools.

165

LEGS AT THE GYM

Working your legs with resistance training is the fastest way to increase metabolism and reduce body fat

Because your legs support your body weight and perform most of the movement you do every day, they are key to changing your body composition. When I suggest doing legs, I have to reinforce that I mean resistance training, not just cardio.

Most people think that cardio exercise is enough work for

their legs. It's not. Cardio and resistance training are two different applications of force and time. Your body responds differently to each one, so even if you are doing cardio, you still need resistance training to build muscle and increase your metabolism. If you do circuit training, you do get a little of both, but when you start to plateau with your results, add

Squats

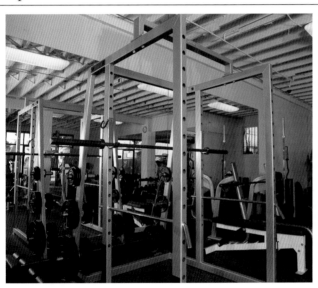

- There are many ways to do squats at the gym: with a free bar, the Smith machine, a ball, or even a leg-press machine.

- Your foot width will depend on your hip width and angle.

- Engage your inner thighs

when you do this exercise so you have more control and stability for the knees and hips.

- Use a small range of motion and light weight to start, and sit your butt behind you to distribute the weight between your hips and knees.

Leg Extension

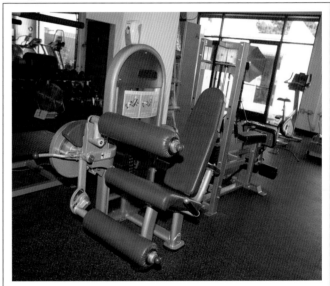

- The leg extension was designed to create resistance and isolate your quadriceps.

- Turn your legs so your kneecaps face the ceiling during the entire exercise.

- Place the bar on your shins as high as is comfortable to minimize the force on your knees. Start with a light weight; visualize activating your quads to lift your lower legs.

- If you have knee problems only use light weights if you can do this pain free.

more focused resistance training before or after your circuit.

The gym usually has some machines that most people do not have at home. Because I teach people the tools they need to work out at home, at the office, or while traveling, when I get into a gym, I use a select few pieces of equipment that I wish I had at home! These are some of my favorite pieces to use when in the gym.

I must also mention body types. If you have the body type that builds muscle quickly—rejoice! A lot of us wish we did, too. I know many women who have this body type are afraid to train their legs for fear of getting too big. While this will not happen for most women, it can for some. Take your measurements, take your body fat, and track it. If you build muscle quickly, maintain the level that you want by not increasing the weight or volume of exercises, but by finding the right amount for you to keep what you have.

Hamstring Curl

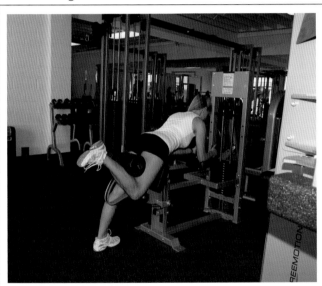

- Working the back of the legs is as important as working the front of the legs; these machines help add resistance.

- The biggest mistake people make using this machine is allowing their hips and butts to move during the exercise.

- Use your glutes to stabilize your hips—this means both your butt and lower back should not move when you do this exercise.

Focus on Lower Body Muscles

- Start with your quadriceps and glutes. They are your largest muscles and a powerhouse of support and strength.

- Work your hamstrings to balance out the strength at your hips and knees and also stretch the quads.

- Adductors and abductors are the muscles on the inside and outside of the hips. Hip strength is critical for long-term strength and balance, and they also stabilize the knees and spine.

- Calves and ankle musculature is best worked in balance exercises. Your feet and ankles are your foundation, and they need to stay strong.

LEG ROUTINES AT HOME
You can do a complete leg workout at home to build muscle without any large equipment

The first question new clients who want to work out at home often ask me is, "Don't I need equipment?" What most people fail to realize is that their body is their equipment! You can use your body weight to create exercises for all parts of your body. Your muscles do not know the difference between a free weight and leg weight—all they know is whether they feel resistance or not. And, when you're ready, you can always increase the difficulty of certain exercises by incorporating a stability ball—a great tool to use when you're working out at home.

Resistance training is about applying force to the muscle that is intense enough to have it fatigue in 45 to 90 seconds.

Standing Hip Flexion

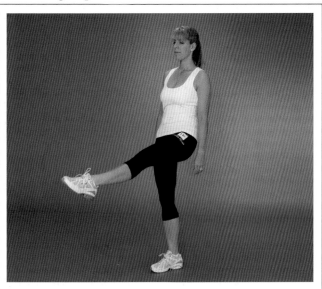

- This exercise works the quadriceps and hip flexors of the moving leg, and it builds hip and ankle stability on the stationary leg.

- People are often surprised by how hard this exercise is for them. The longer your leg, the harder it is.

- You can do this exercise anywhere and repeat it three times on each leg for a good start to a great leg workout.

- See "Beginner Resistance" in Chapter 16 for complete instructions on how to do this exercise.

Ball Squats

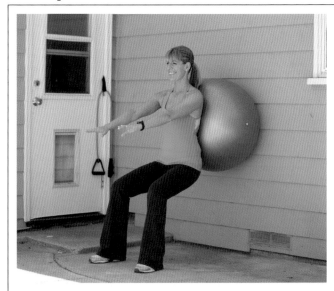

- The ball allows you to adjust your form to fit your body, and because the ball helps hold you up, it's a better choice than a freestanding squat.

- Balls come in three sizes: 55, 65, and 75 centimeters. Choose a ball that reflects your height. Are you small, medium, or large?

- You can hold free weights in your hands to make this exercise harder.

- See "Intermediate Resistance" in Chapter 17 for instructions on how to do this exercise.

How you apply that resistance does not matter when it comes to building muscles. How you apply resistance will be important for the health and longevity of your joints, but the muscles inside your body only feel it as enough resistance or not enough. The gym has some great tools, but what do you do when you travel or cannot get to the gym? Here are a few exercises you can do to work your legs at home.

Prone Hip Extension

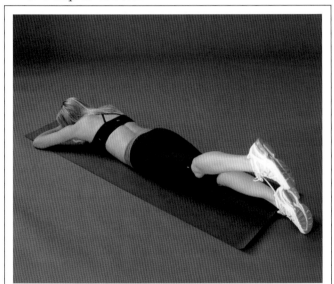

- This is a standard hamstring and glute exercise that you can do anywhere.

- The longer your leg, the more difficult the exercise. Start with a small range of motion and increase slowly.

- The range of motion for this exercise is not large

- anyway; it becomes more of a lower back exercise if you go too high.

- You can use an ankle weight to increase the intensity when you need it.

- See "Intermediate Resistance" in Chapter 17 for instructions.

Ball Bridge or Bridge

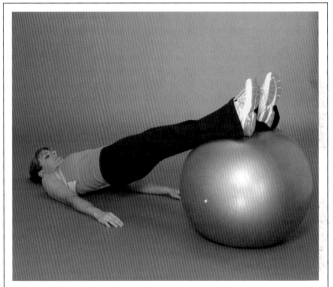

- The bridge is a great exercise for stretching the quads and hip flexors.

- If you use a ball, you can push the ball farther away from you toward your feet to make it harder.

- You can also pull the ball in toward your knee to make it easier, as more of your body weight is supported by the ball.

- See "Advanced Resistance" in Chapter 17 for complete instructions on how to do this exercise.

IT ALL COUNTS!

UPPER BODY AT THE GYM

A variety of exercises and types of resistance can make for an interesting upper-body workout

I think I prefer doing upper body at the gym because of the variety of exercises and forms of resistance available. But I also know that a lot of women are intimidated by all the machines in a regular gym when they don't know how to use them. We discuss form a lot in this book, so I hope you will apply what you've learned to the exercises you do at home

and at the gym to build your confidence.

If you attend a women-only gym, you may or may not have access to some of these pieces of equipment. It is important to work the upper body to maintain bone health, muscle strength, and appearance (of course) and to avoid common injuries while doing normal everyday activities caused by

Chest Press on Cable Cross

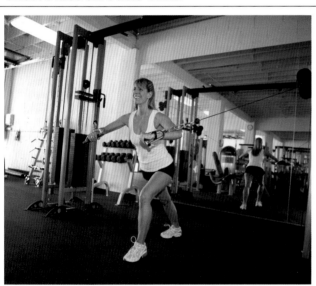

- I love cables because you can angle yourself and the cables to fit your body and your motion.

- You can also do a chest exercise in an upright position. You do most chest exercises on your back because you use gravity.

- Your muscles work differently with cables, because you do not have to deal with inertia. Aim for smooth, slow movements and control in both directions.

- See "Intermediate Resistance" in Chapter 17 for complete instructions.

Chest Press on Incline Bench

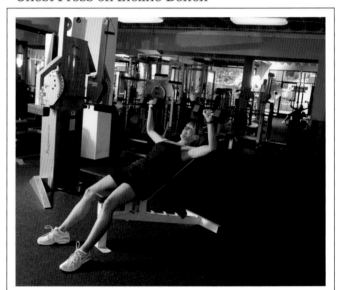

- If you don't have an incline bench, you can lie on a mat or on a ball.

- Changing the angle changes the motor pattern, so you may be able to activate muscles in your chest and shoulders that you are not able to in other exercises.

- When you raise the back of the bench to become more vertical, you activate more shoulder and less chest muscle. Aim for a 30-degree incline as your average starting point.

lack of strength. Doing upper-body exercises will not make a drastic change in your metabolism, but you will probably see changes in the mirror faster than you do with lower–body exercises.

Muscles you want to work on include chest, back, shoulders, biceps, triceps, and forearms and hands (grip strength) and muscles of the spine and lower back. Even though you are using machines, use your own body and abs to support and stabilize you as your do these exercises.

Seated Row

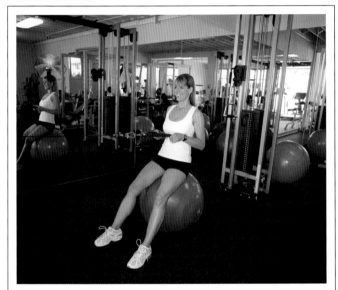

- When doing back exercises, make sure to engage your back before your arms; otherwise it becomes an arm exercise.

- There are machines specifically for this exercise that have a chest pad—try not to use that. You can also create a row with added core involvement by using a ball at a cable machine.

- Keep your feet flat on the ground; use the ground and your foundation to help you.

- See "Intermediate Resistance" in Chapter 17 for instructions.

Lat Pull Down

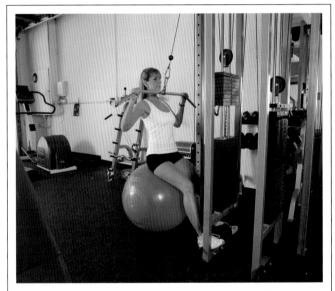

- Place your arms as wide as your shoulders on the bar, then use your shoulder blades to initiate pulling the bar down toward your chest.

- Use your back muscles and then your arm muscles to pull your shoulder blades together.

- Your focus should not be on the bar to the chest but the shoulder blades down and together.

- A myth about the lat pull down is that it works different parts of the muscle if you use a wide grip versus a narrow grip.

IT ALL COUNTS!

UPPER BODY AT HOME

Use tools you already have to create an upper-body workout at home

Most people have a few fitness gadgets at home, such as a mat or a ball or even a piece of tubing or a set of small free weights. When you start creating exercises for your upper body at home, you do not need very much to start. When you learn the correct form and variations of exercises you can do anywhere, you start looking at the world differently.

I see a stairway as an exercise tool. It's a piece of cardio equipment that can also help with resistance training. I can create one exercise on it, or I can spend 20 to 30 minutes getting a great workout, which would include cardio and resistance. I see a short wall between beach properties as a ledge to do a push-up on. I see a lamppost or a tree as an anchor

Push-Up

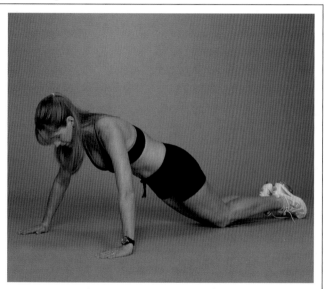

- The push-up is a classic upper-body exercise you can do anywhere.

- It works mostly the shoulders and triceps, with some chest and abs, too. If you have shoulder problems, start with plank to strengthen and activate your shoulder muscles.

- This is exercise is simple to make easier or harder for any level. You can do it against a wall or on a mat. Start with 5 to 10 and see how you do.

Chest Press on Mat

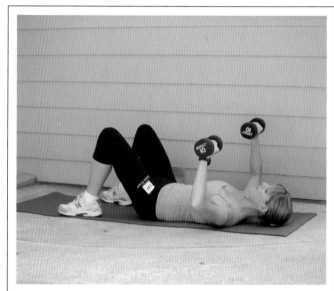

- The easiest place to start a chest press is on a mat.

- This exercise can help train you to not let your arms go any farther than 90 degrees, since you would hit the floor.

- Most women start off with too little weight. Learn the motion and start with at least 5 pounds until you feel comfortable; then increase.

- See "Intermediate Resistance" in Chapter 17 for instructions.

for my exercise tubing. Even if you have no gadgets, you can create a beginner exercise program for your upper body. On these pages I will introduce you to a few of my favorite exercises I do at home or at the beach. I hope you can try them out soon and feel how easy it is to exercise anywhere.

Row

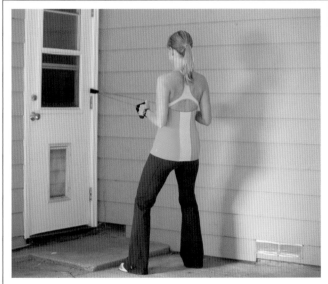

- This exercise requires some tubing, a doorstop, and a door that you can anchor the tubing to. You could also wrap the tubing around a pole or tree.

- Concentrate on using your back muscles while standing up. Spend your energy focused on the exercise, not your posture.

- This works the lats, traps, rhomboids, rear deltoids, and biceps.

- See "Intermediate Resistance" in Chapter 17 for instructions.

Rear Delt Row

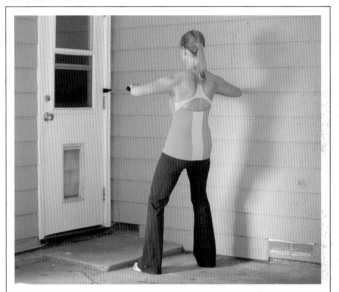

- This exercise targets the back of the shoulder, the back of the neck, the traps, and the biceps.

- You will feel your shoulders working the most because they are holding your arms in the air so you can do the exercise.

- If you do not have a doorstop to help anchor the tubing, a tree, pole, or handrail on the stairs may work, too.

- See "Advanced Resistance" in Chapter 17 for instructions.

IT ALL COUNTS!

THE DIET

Much of your success in changing your body depends on what you eat each day

People often think diet is more important than exercise when it comes to weight loss, and it is on some levels. Food is the body's fuel system and eating is how you get the nutrients your body needs to stay healthy. With a proper diet, exercise can make a significant difference, but exercise alone cannot erase the damage caused by a poor diet.

Eliminate or reduce any processed or packaged foods you eat. They may be convenient and taste good, but they are usually filled with preservatives, chemicals, high-fructose corn syrup, and other ingredients that can elevate insulin and blood sugar and clog your arteries and are toxic for your liver.

If you feel tired often and crave more energy, change your

Lean Protein

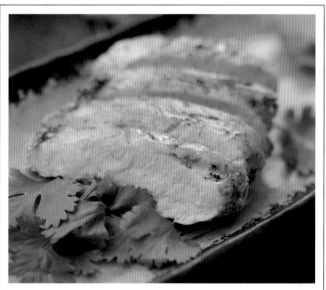

- Your meal should center around a protein choice.

- Fish, eggs, meat, tofu, and tempeh are all great protein choices. Depending on your size, aim for 4 to 6 ounces or at least 15 to 20 grams of protein.

- Most protein choices are versatile enough to have at breakfast, lunch, or dinner and even as a snack.

- You can also substitute a protein shake for a meal when you're on the go or want something easy.

Colorful Fruits and Veggies

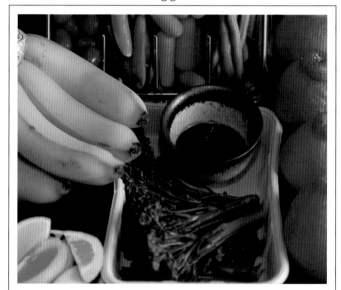

- Aim to get color into your diet through veggies and fruit.

- Make it a goal to eat the rainbow every day, and alternate the things you choose for each color every few days.

- Aim to have 1 cup of fruits

- and/or veggies at breakfast and 2 cups at lunch and dinner every day.

- If you can find a local farmers' market or even grow your own fruits and veggies, you'll have more nutrient-rich foods that come straight from the soil to your plate.

diet to fresh, live foods, not chemical-laden versions of fresh food. Start by making a food log to help you determine which changes you are willing to make. Cut down on or eliminate going to drive-thrus and eating fast and fried foods. Replace soda with water—or sparkling water with some freshly squeezed juice. Most people understand healthy choices on some level, so ask yourself what three things you are willing to change right now.

Healthy Fats

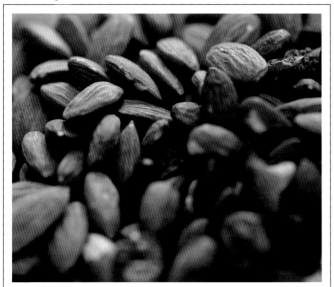

- Nuts are a great way to get healthy fats into your diet.

- Other healthy fats include avocado, olive oil, coconut, and the fat found in fish.

- Fat does not make you fat, so make sure you have some in each meal. You need it for your brain, organs, and cells.

- If you love your butter and cheese, enjoy them, but try not to eat too much of them. They are higher in saturated fat.

Starch

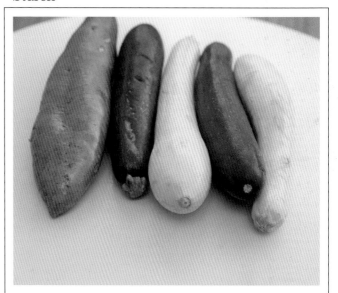

- Get your starch from sources like sweet potatoes, yams, potatoes, and squash.

- Brown and white rice are easy for the body to digest for most people.

- Limit your starch intake to once a day, if possible, and eat it at the meal before the time of day when you are most active. That way you can use those calories as energy right away.

- Choose starches with high fiber to keep you satisfied longer and help your digestive system move things along.

AB ROUTINE

This beginner routine for the abs will fully engage your entire core

In exercise, just as in sports, it's always good to start with the basics. Creating a good foundation for the progression of your exercise routine and body sets up a strong platform from which to grow. Too many people leap from being sedentary to being highly active, and then they get injured or frustrated. I see this happen over and over again. It is almost like an addiction when people throw themselves into a new lifestyle, get great results, and then plateau and lose the momentum because of unrealistic expectations. They usually fall backward again—back to the beginning or worse.

Start by doing 1 set of each of these exercises every day. On the third or fourth exercise day, if they are getting easy or are not hard enough on the second day, increase to 2 sets of each exercise in the order listed here. When that becomes too easy, increase to 3 sets of each exercise for a few weeks before progressing to the intermediate level. Be sure that you

Isometric in Tabletop

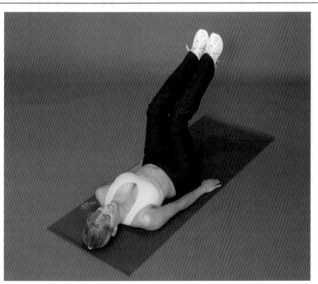

- When doing your beginner ab routine, start with this exercise.

- We covered isometrics in detail in Chapter 9; review that chapter for more details on how to properly perform this exercise.

- Hold this position with your back firmly on the ground for 60 seconds to start.

- Do 3 sets in a row, taking 60 to 90 seconds of rest in between. If 60 seconds is too much, do 3 sets of 45 seconds each and work your way up.

Half Crunch Upper

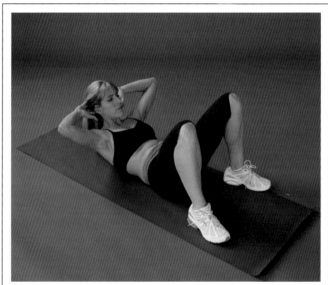

- We covered this exercise in Chapter 10; review that chapter for cues for doing it properly.

- Move slowly and lift yourself up for 2 seconds and lower yourself back down for 2 seconds. Do not rest for long between reps.

- Start with 1 to 3 sets of 20 to 30 reps after you complete the isometric in tabletop ab exercise above. This is the second exercise.

do the exercise slowly and do not stop moving until the set it over. Limit your rest in between sets to 60 seconds or less and if you need to challenge yourself more, do more reps until you fatigue.

Half-Bicycle

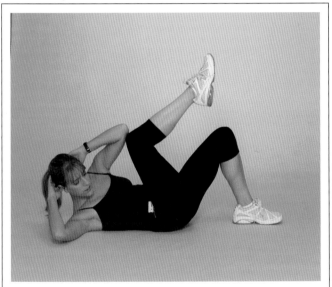

- For more detailed instructions on how to properly do this exercise, refer back to Chapter 11.

- The half-bicycle allows you to connect your brain to your obliques, so it is important to establish the motor pattern before adding more resistance.

- Do each rep with a 4-second rep speed—2 counts up and 2 counts down. Each side counts as 1 rep. Exhale as you lift off the ground.

- Start with 1 to 3 sets of 40 repetitions.

Single Leg Pull

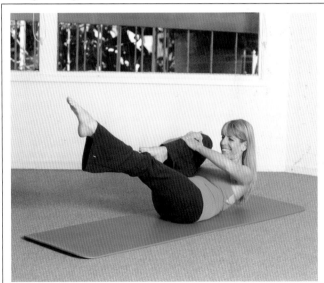

- Refer to Chapter 13 for instructions on how to achieve proper form and technique for Pilates.

- This is the hardest exercise in this series for beginners. I put it at the end so that all your core muscles will have been engaged before doing this exercise.

- You can time this for 60 seconds, or you can count each leg pull as 1 rep. In that case, do 30 reps, holding each for 2 seconds and do 1 to 3 sets.

CARDIO PLAN

Choose cardiovascular activities that you have easy access to and fit your current fitness level

When beginners get started, the biggest complaint I hear is that they don't like to exercise or that it's really hard. Remember that you do not have to put in a certain amount of time or even effort to get started—just get started. You can also add more movement into your life by simply taking the stairs instead of the elevator and parking your car farther away

from your destination than you might be used to. I once had someone follow all my suggestions and implement all these little steps 1 month before she even started her exercise program, and she lost 10 pounds in 30 days with minimal effort.

Think of three ways you can get more movement into your day and then do them. Commit to some focused cardio that

Treadmill

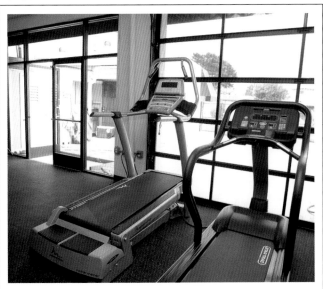

- The treadmill is one of the most popular pieces of home exercise equipment. If you do not have one or easy access to one, you can substitute walking.

- Because walking on the treadmill is very close to a movement we already do, it is normally not very chal-

lenging to start a walking cardio program.

- Aim to walk briskly using your arms for 10 to 15 minutes to start. If this is easy, increase your pace and your time.

Outdoor Bike

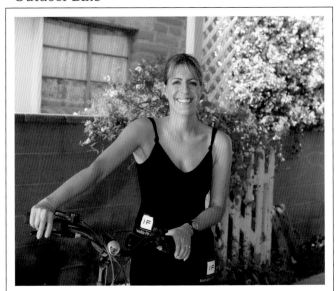

- An outdoor bike is another easy way to get some cardio.

- Because a bike holds your body weight for you, riding is easier on the body in general.

- Unless you are doing some hills or climbing a bit, your

heart rate might not get as high riding a bike as walking on a treadmill, so consider riding for a longer duration.

- Use a bike for transportation. My husband and I now bike instead of drive to dinner at a local restaurant.

you can somewhat easily fit into your schedule. If you are a super-busy person who is unwilling to make time, find 10 minutes to start either at the beginning or end of your day, and that is where you will put your cardio for now.

In this first 7 days, try one or all of the exercises listed below and plan to do at least 15 to 30 minutes of exercise each day if your schedule allows. If you want faster results, you can do cardio every day or every other day.

MAKE IT EASY

The cardio suggestions listed here are ones that I have found to be easily accessible for most people and easy on the body for anyone with joint concerns. They also can be done almost anywhere. Feel free to add your favorite cardio activities if I have not listed them. Any repetitive action that gets your heart rate elevated for more than 10 minutes is considered cardio.

Dancing

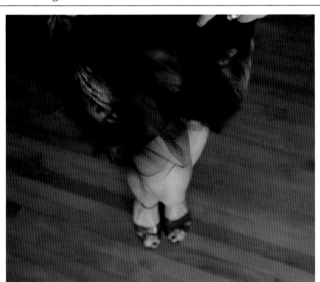

- Most women have music they love to listen to that inspires then to move. Your favorite music can be a very powerful tool for you.

- If you do not like dancing in public, put on your favorite music, close the shades, and dance around for 10 to 15 minutes.

- If you have always dreamed of learning to dance, sign up for a dance class.

- If you are a trained dancer, work it back into your life.

Cardio Basics

- Make a commitment to do some focused cardio at least once to four times every week for 4 to 6 weeks.

- Choose exercises that are easy to do and that you have easy access to. Pick your favorite movement first to inspire you to do it more often.

- Experiment with different kinds of cardio to find what works for you.

- Get your heart rate up to a level where you cannot have a smooth conversation.

BEGINNER RESISTANCE

A simple four-step exercise plan can get any beginner started with total-body resistance training

The excuse I hear most often for not exercising is lack of time. A close second is a dislike for going to the gym. Well, you do not need to go to the gym if you don't want to. This beginner routine I put together consists of four exercises that incorporate many of the major muscle groups, and it can be done in 30 minutes or less at home or anywhere you like! If resistance training and the gym intimidate you, start with these exercises you can do at home. If you say you do not have time, you can do this routine while you watch a 30-minute television program—it's that easy.

These exercises are simple yet effective at starting to help you build muscle. There are many levels to progress to and

Standing Hip Flexion

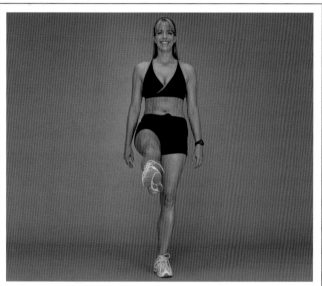

- Stand with feet hip width apart and body weight shifted to your left.

- Point the right toe, lock the right knee, and imagine pulling your leg off the ground by using your quads.

- Do not throw or kick your leg.

- Lift slowly for 2 counts and lower for 2 without resting at the bottom. Start with 2 to 3 sets of 20 to 25 reps on each leg.

Bridge

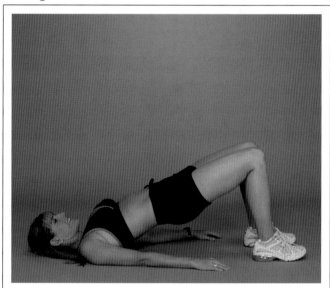

- Lie on your back with your knees bent and feet flat on the ground.

- Imagine moving the muscles from the back of your knee to your lower back.

- Lift yourself off the ground when your hamstring contracts, and move 2 counts

in each direction as you lift and lower; do not rest on the floor between reps.

- Start with 3 sets of 25 to 30 reps. You should feel the contraction in your glutes and hamstrings and a stretch in your quads.

there are hundreds of exercises to choose from. I chose these because they are simple and can be done anywhere, so you have no excuse! If you are somewhere without free weights, you can use exercise tubing, soup cans, or anything you have two of that weighs 3 to 8 pounds.

As you build strength with these exercises, you will also gain flexibility. You may be surprised to find your flexibility increase from resistance training. It's actually what should happen with a well-designed balanced program. Do 1 to 3 sets of each of these exercises every other day in your first 7 days.

Plank on Knees

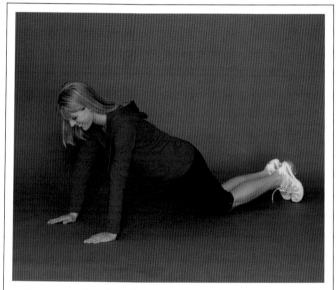

- Get on your hands and knees with arms shoulder width apart.

- Place a pillow under your knees to cushion them against the floor.

- Transfer most of your body weight to your arms and hold this position. Keep your abs tight; make sure to breathe.

- Hold for 60 seconds and do 3 sets in a row. If this is too easy, you can stretch your legs behind you and do it on your toes; hold for 30 to 45 seconds to start.

Shoulder Press

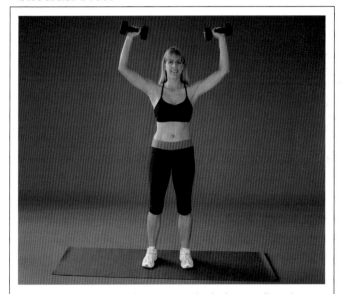

- You can do this seated or standing. Start with light weights, around 5 or 8 pounds.

- With your arms bent in a 90-degree angle over your shoulders, lift the weights up and over your head.

- Think about pulling the deltoids from the outside of the arms to the center of your body instead of pushing, so you can activate the muscle better.

- Start with 2 to 3 sets of 20 to 25 reps and adjust the weight or reps to fit your fitness level.

SLEEP

Getting enough sleep is as important as exercise for weight loss

Have you heard you can sleep yourself thin? You can, and I will explain. There are hundreds of thousands of people in the world who live highly stressful lives and get little to no sleep. What do you think that does to the body? Why do we need sleep?

Sleep is the time the body needs to rest, replenish, renew, and grow. When you work out, your muscles need recovery time. You do not build muscle while you use it, your body builds it while you sleep and are at rest.

Your body also needs to replenish other things, too, including hormones. Cortisol is one of the adrenal hormones; if you recall, it's the body's "fight or flight" hormone. Imagine living in a "fight or flight" state all the time. It would be exhausting and taxing on the body. Not having enough sleep is a serious problem for your adrenal hormones, your focus and concentration, and your immune system. Burnout in medical terms

Hot Bubble Bath

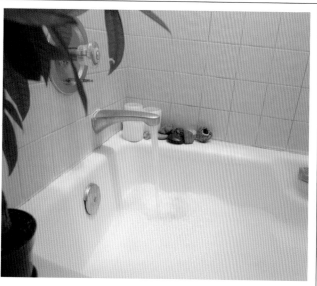

- A bath is a great way to unwind at the end of a day. You can add so many things to a bath to help you relax.

- From lavender bath salts to Epsom salts, there are many products that offer stress relief through aromatherapy.

- Essential oils are great in a bath too, because they offer different healing properties. Lavender helps you to relax, while peppermint stimulates the brain.

Tea and a Journal

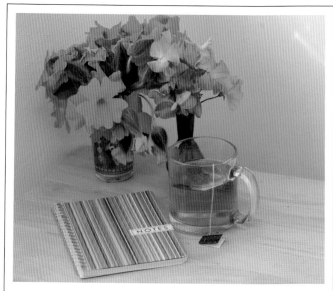

- If you don't have time every night for a bath, at least make some time to sip caffeine-free tea.

- There are many herbal teas to choose from depending on your taste.

- If you don't like tea, hot lemon water can work, too.

Stay away from high-sugar hot drinks like cocoa or apple cider before bed, because they can spike your blood sugar.

- Keep a journal close by and practice unloading any last thoughts of the day before drifting off to sleep.

is called adrenal fatigue, and it can make losing weight and building muscle very hard for your body.

If you are having a hard time losing weight, and you don't sleep well, I encourage you to work on this immediately. Practice unwinding at the end of your day before you go to sleep. Avoid sugar and caffeine after seven o'clock and drink plenty of water. Look for ways to improve your sleep naturally before resorting to medication. Try the evening relaxation meditation from my 6 Week Beach Body Program for free (see Chapter 20). It's a 17-minute hypnosis that you listen to every night before bed to help you sleep. Our clients rave about it and enjoy deeper, more restful sleep.

Meditation

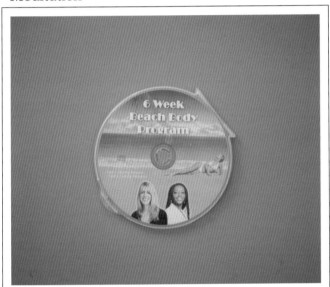

- I also use creative visualization and meditation to help people change their stress levels naturally.

- Sometimes the stress that is driving you starts with underlying thoughts and feelings in your subconscious mind.

- There are many hypnosis programs on the market as well as hypnotherapists who can help you one-on-one if you desire.

- Hypnosis a great tool that is very effective in helping people release stress and sleep better.

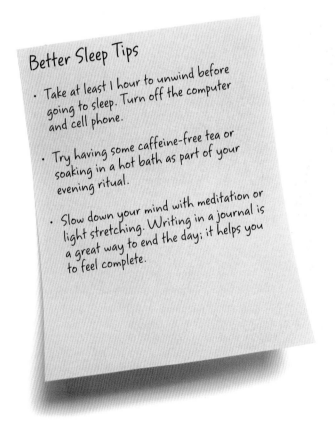

Better Sleep Tips

- Take at least 1 hour to unwind before going to sleep. Turn off the computer and cell phone.

- Try having some caffeine-free tea or soaking in a hot bath as part of your evening ritual.

- Slow down your mind with meditation or light stretching. Writing in a journal is a great way to end the day; it helps you to feel complete.

SUPPLEMENTS

Taking at least a few vitamins every day can make a big difference in your health

Because most of us do not get the nutrition we need from our food, I encourage the use of vitamin and mineral supplements. Even though food should be the first way to try to get all of your nutrients, the depletion of nutrients in the soil, the shelf life of produce, and the chemicals used in mass farming all make it difficult to get all the vitamins and minerals our bodies need. So most of us need to take supplements to help our bodies achieve optimum levels of nutrition. However, there are so many supplements on the market that it can be overwhelming to choose one if you don't know what you should be taking. It is a good idea to identify your specific needs and avoid taking unnecessary supplements.

Omega-3s/Krill Oil

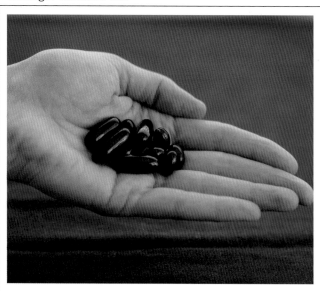

- If you were to take only one supplement, this is the one I would recommend.

- First, they help to lower cholesterol and help fight heart disease.

- Second, fish oil is a natural anti-inflammatory and can help with general inflam-

mation or injuries.

- Fish oil is good for brain health and can help you sleep, because it calms the nervous system.

- There have been reports of fish oil helping with weight loss. Aim for at least 2,000 mg a day.

Vitamin D

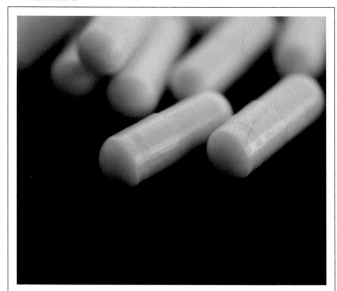

- You need vitamin D to maintain normal blood levels of calcium and phosphorus.

- Recent research suggests vitamin D may provide protection from osteoporosis, high blood pressure, cancer, depression, diabetes, obesity, and other diseases.

- To be sure you get enough vitamin D, get a blood test. If you are low, you can take a supplement.

- Aim to get 5,000 IU of vitamin D as a preventive measure for the long list of conditions mentioned.

I can make a few recommendations across the board based on research that suggests most of our diets lack certain important nutrients. And rest assured that I would not recommend anything I do not take myself. But before you invest in any supplements, talk to your alternative medicine doctor or registered dietician about their recommended brands. As with any other product, not all supplements are made the same. Some contain cheap fillers and have a lower absorption rate.

YELLOW LIGHT

I am not an expert on supplements, so I encourage you to consult with the medical people in your life whom you trust or to find a registered dietician or alternative medicine doctor who is aware of current research on supplementation. I have listed four of the supplements I take each day that offer vitamins for most of the major functions of the body and are needed by most Americans.

Probiotics

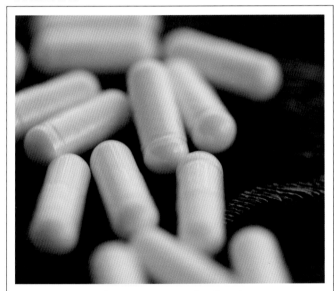

- Digestive issues have become more common, especially among people who have difficulty losing weight.

- Probiotics are the good bacteria that live in the digestive system; they help break down foods so you can digest them more easily.

- The digestive system controls up to 80 percent of your immune system, so having healthy digestion can affect your overall health.

- Probiotics come in many forms—find one that works for you.

Vitamin C/Antioxidants

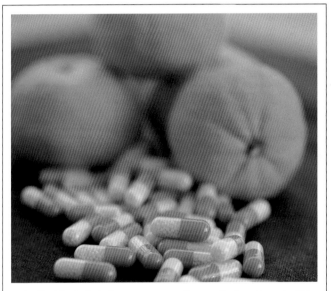

- Antioxidants help keep you healthy and young by fighting off the effects of free radicals that lead to cell death.

- Free radicals are like the exhaust from a car. The body makes them naturally, but they are also in the environment.

- Free radicals can cause premature aging, like rust on a car, if you lack antioxidants to fight them off.

- Antioxidants occur naturally in fruits and veggies, green tea, dark chocolate, and red wine.

INTERMEDIATE ABS

Progressing to the next level with your abs means increasing the intensity of the exercises

Once you have become comfortable with the beginner exercises, learned the movements, and established a connection between your brain and the muscles, it's time to add more intensity.

You will move from lifting the lighter half of your body to lifting the heavier half of your body. You will practice using both your upper and lower body as resistance at the same time. If this routine is a larger jump than you are ready for, feel free to mix and match a few exercises from the beginner and intermediate routines. Know your body and learn to listen to it.

You will notice as you progress and get stronger that you

Half Crunch Lower

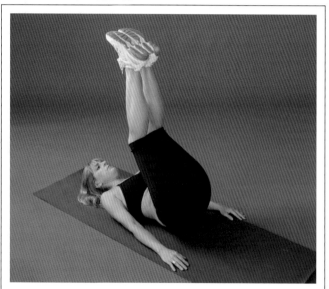

- It is time to progress to lifting more of your body weight with your abs.

- See Chapter 10 for instructions on how to do this exercise.

- Start by doing 2 to 3 sets of 20 to 25 reps slowly; make sure not to swing your legs or use momentum.

- You do not need to start off with a large range of motion. Do what you can and watch how you improve. The longer or thicker your legs are, the more resistance you have in this exercise.

Ball Crunch

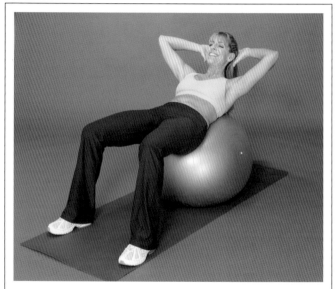

- Try adding some instability to the regular crunch.

- You can find instructions on how to do abs on the ball in Chapter 12.

- Start where you can comfortably let your upper body lower over the ball while stabilizing yourself with your feet.

- Try 2 to 3 sets of 25 to 30 reps; do them slowly and with good form. If you want to make the work harder, walk your body farther off the ball so your abs have to pull up more of your upper body.

can do more. You may feel the exercise differently, whether it be that you can sense more of your muscles working while exercising or you feel a different kind of soreness in your muscles in the days following your workout. Pay attention to what your body is telling you. If you feel nothing at all on the days after your workouts, you may not be working hard enough. When you progress to intermediate level, start with 2 sets of each exercise every other day and increase to 3 sets as the work gets easier.

Bicycle

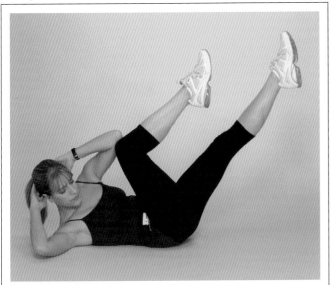

- The challenge with the full bicycle is that both your upper and lower body offer resistance to your abs at the same time.

- For instructions on how to do this exercise with proper form, review Chapter 11.

- Start with 2 to 3 sets of 30 to 40 reps, counting each side as 1 rep.

- Make sure to do this exercise slowly; concentrate on your abs pulling your body into the center, not on throwing your arms or legs.

Single Leg Stretch

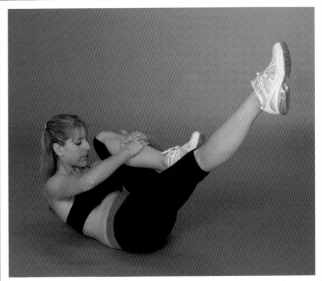

- This exercise is the next level of progression after the single leg pull; see Chapter 13 for instructions.

- Start with 2 to 3 sets of 30 reps, counting each side as 1 and taking 2 counts for each leg.

- If you need some neck support, trying doing this exercise with one hand behind your head. If that is not enough, you can keep your head on the ground and only focus on the lower part.

INTERMEDIATE CARDIO

Intermediate cardio will be slightly more intense—it is also time to understand heart rate

Intermediate cardio can be created from any of the exercises I mention here, or even in the beginners' list of cardio activities. What separates the beginner from the intermediate exerciser when it comes to cardio is the commitment to doing the exercises and the time spent understanding and tracking the heart rate.

My mother was a seasoned walker, but she swore she would never run. For years and years she kept off her weight and got some exercise by walking. But eventually she wanted to get to a new level, so we used a heart rate monitor to track how hard and efficiently she was working. Most of the women like my mother, who have been walking for years, find out that

Jogging

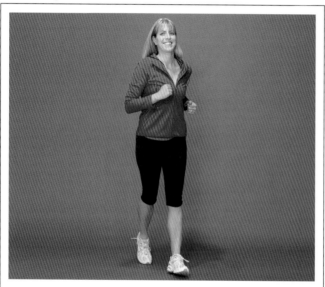

- The difference between walking and jogging can be as simple as a small bounce.

- Rather than taking long strides with a walk, keep your feet underneath you and add a small bounce.

- Jogging can range from very slow to fast. Find a comfortable pace that is a small step up from a fast walk.

- Try 10 to 15 minutes to start, or put a few minutes of jogging in between 3 to 5 minutes of fast walking to get you started.

Elliptical

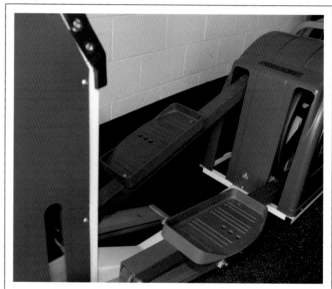

- The elliptical trainer is a great machine for several reasons. It is the only machine you can go backward on safely.

- Going backward is a whole new motor pattern for your body and can help activate new muscle fibers.

- Elliptical trainers are great for people with knee issues, because they do not have a lot of impact.

- Start with 20 or 30 minutes on a manual setting and see how it feels. As you progress, add resistance by increasing the level, if necessary.

their exercise helps them maintain their weight but it does not help them to lose weight, because they are not working at a level that will produce change.

Once my mother started using her heart rate monitor, she found she had to jog, because it was the only way for her to get in her target heart rate zone, where she would receive some benefit. (See pages 194 and 195 for more on target heart rate.) Her walking was good for her overall health, but it was not offering enough intensity to cause physical changes.

Being at this level means it is time to get a heart rate monitor and know exactly what your body is doing and how hard you are working.

Once you progress to intermediate cardio, you are increasing your intensity for more results, so replace your cardio choice with one of those listed on these pages. You can also increase your duration to at least 30 to 60 minutes every other day or every day depending on your goals.

Jump Rope

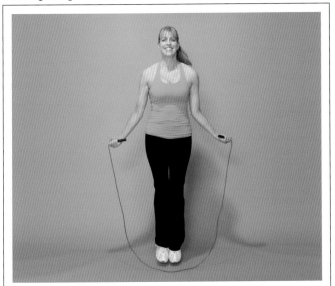

- I put jumping rope in the intermediate program because it can be effective in short intervals.

- You can do a single or double bounce, and you can start by counting how many you can do in a row.

- This is a great exercise to build your calves.

- Start counting how many you can do and then progress from that number. This is a much more intense exercise, but I am not suggesting you do it for 15 to 20 minutes straight at this level.

Jumping Jacks

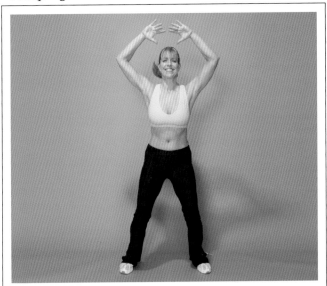

- Because of the impact, make sure your body can handle doing jumping jacks by starting off with a small number.

- For correct form for both jumping rope and jumping jacks, review Chapter 8. Start on carpet or grass so you have more cushion.

- Start with 30 or 40 reps and see how you feel. Do 2 or 3 sets with a minute rest in between.

- Use both jumping exercises to enhance a walk or a lower-level cardio activity to make it harder.

INTERMEDIATE RESISTANCE

Adding extra resistance with tubing and dumbbells is the next step for intermediate resistance training

The exercises I'm suggesting on these pages cover most of the major muscle groups. The squat targets the quads, glutes, and calves, while the prone hip extension works the hamstrings and glutes and stretches the hip flexors and quads. The chest press works the chest, shoulders, and triceps, while the row works the back muscles and the biceps.

If you have only 30 minutes to do an exercise program, these are the exercises I would recommend for a well-rounded full-body program.

When it comes to the squat with a ball, I am a strong supporter that exercisers find the right form based on their own bodies and not by simply following or mimicing someone

Squat with a Ball

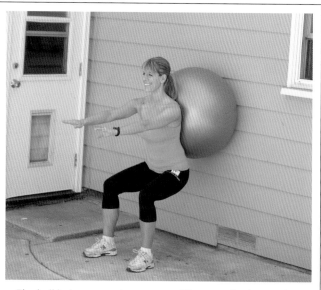

- The ball helps prevent feeling pain or discomfort in your knees and back in a squat.

- Place the ball on the wall behind you at your lower back level and walk your feet out in front of you.

- Allow your body to sit back behind you as if you were sitting in a chair. Adjust your feet placement and amount of flexion in your hips and knees to a place that feels comfortable.

- Start with 2 to 3 sets of 30 to 35 reps.

Prone Hip Extension

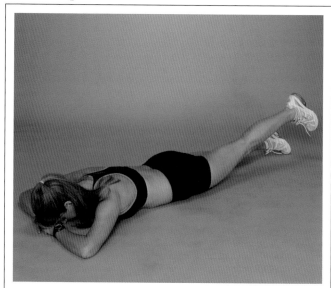

- Lie facedown on the floor. Put your forehead on your hands and relax your shoulders and neck.

- Exhale as you lift your left leg off the ground with your hamstring and glutes. You work one leg at a time.

- This can start as a short

range of motion, which should only increase when you feel you can pull more with the back of your leg.

- Start with 2 to 3 sets of 25 to 30 reps slowly using 2 counts up and 2 counts down; do not rest your leg on the ground between reps.

else's form. The ball allows you to make adjustments because you can change the placement of your feet, and how much of your body sits back behind them. I recommend the squat with a ball over a freestanding squat for most people because we each have a unique body; the form that's right for one person may not be right for the next.

The workout below can be done in 25 to 30 minutes with 3 sets per exercise. When you increase to intermediate, be sure to do these exercises in the order they are listed here, 2 to 3 sets each, every other day.

As an intermediate exerciser, you can begin to work more with tubing. It's lightweight, travels well, and can generate enough resistance for a good workout for most people. You will need a doorstop or anchor to do the row exercise, unless you have a tree or pole to wrap the tubing around. Some brands sell an anchor or doorstop with their tubing.

Chest Press

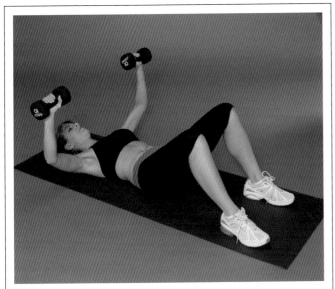

- Lie on your back with your knees bent. Holding light weights (5 to 10 pounds) in each hand, extend your arms over your chest.

- Lower your arms out and down until you create a right angle in your arms. Your elbows lead the

motion as you lower the weights.

- Pull your arms up and together over your chest and bring the weights together.

- Do 2 to 3 sets of 30 to 35 reps very slowly.

Row or One Arm Row

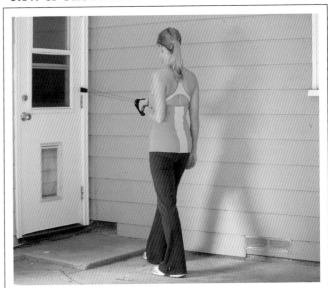

- This is one of the most important exercises women can do to help with their posture and back strength.

- Secure the tubing in front of you with a height between your chest and shoulder level.

- Grab the handles in your

hands and step back. Using two arms is easier than using one. This is the advanced version but the form is the same.

- Initiate the movement with your shoulder blades. Start with a medium-thickness resistance band and do 2 to 3 sets of 30 to 35 reps.

191

ADVANCED ABS

These advanced exercises use both your upper and lower body weight as resistance for every exercise

When you get to the advanced level for abs, you use more resistance than you do in the first two levels. If you feel you are more advanced than intermediate, but these exercises are too difficult for you at this time, either adjust them or start with one at a time. You may want to mix and match exercises from all three sections to add volume to your workout.

Advanced exercisers are generally people who work out often and have increased their strength beyond the exercises suggested for the beginner or intermediate exerciser. None of these levels indicates anything about results or health, only strength. You may be an advanced exerciser but feel that you have a long way to go with your goals, which may

Advanced Bicycle

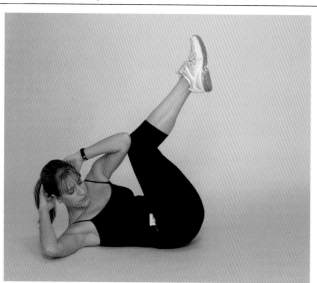

- For detailed instructions on how to do this exercise, refer to Chapter 11.

- The slower you do most exercises, the harder they become. Aim to do this one slowly with complete control.

- Start with 2 to 3 sets of 30

reps, counting each side as 1 and taking 2 seconds to pull in and 2 seconds to return to neutral before going to the other side.

- I placed this exercise first, because I want you to have all your energy and focus to do this exercise with control.

Full Crunch

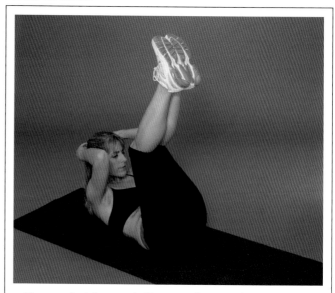

- You may find that one half of your body moves more than the other. This is normal. Consult Chapter 5 for instructions.

- You want to focus on moving both sides of your body into the center. If you have long legs, your lower body may have a greater range

of motion than your upper body.

- Start with 3 sets of 25 to 30 reps; do them very slowly and concentrate on your abs doing all the work.

- At an advanced level, you need more volume, so progress to 3 sets.

have nothing or everything to do with exercise. Use this book to review your entire fitness and weight-loss plan.

When you move on to the advanced level, you may want to add these exercises to the intermediate routine and work the upper and lower body in two separate workouts. As you progress, you also need more volume per muscle group, not just greater intensity. Aim to do the combined upper body routine twice a week and the combined lower body twice a week.

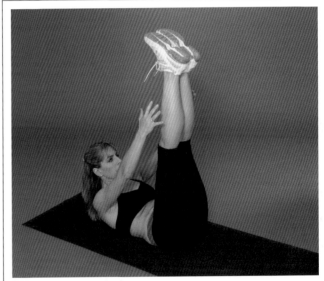
JJ's Ball Pass

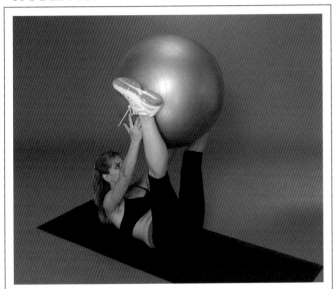

- Just as in the full crunch, one side of your body may have more range of motion than the other. Just make sure to focus on pulling both sides in as much as you can. Consult Chapter 12 for instructions.

- Start with 2 to 3 sets of 25 to 30 reps, counting each crunch as a rep regardless of where the ball is.

- If holding the ball makes this too difficult because your legs are not strong enough yet, use a pillow so you can focus on your abs first.

Double Leg Stretch

- This is the hardest of the Pilates ab exercises that I have included here; it is definitely an advanced exercise. Consult Chapter 13 for instructions.

- You use all your body weight in the longest position possible, and this will generate the most amount of resistance with your body weight.

- Start with 2 or 3 sets of 10 to 15 reps. It's more important to do a few of these with perfect form than to do more with poor form.

193

ADVANCED CARDIO

Advanced cardio can mean working your full body for maximum calorie burning

It's time to calculate your target heart rate zone. The formula I use is the Karvonen Formula: 220 - age - resting heart rate = X. To find your resting heart rate (RHR), use your first two fingers to find your pulse on your wrist or neck. Take this reading before you get out of bed in the morning. Count the first pulse you feel as 0 and then count 1, 2, and so on. Count the

beats for 6 seconds and then add a 0 to that number. For example, if you count 7 beats, your RHR is approximately 70. Next, plug your RHR into the formula to find X, and then multiply X times the percentages you want to use to establish your target heart rate zone. Some people use 50 to 85 percent as their zone. I think 50 percent is too low, so I start with

Boxing

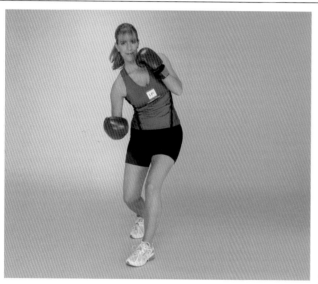

- For details on form, review "Boxing" in Chapter 6.

- There are easy ways to do boxing as your cardio, even if you do not have a gym or heavy bag. Shadow boxing is throwing the punches without hitting something and can be done anywhere.

- There are also standing bags you fill with water or sand and can move around inside or out.

- Start with 20 to 30 minutes of continuous boxing moves with some music for an advanced cardio workout.

Kickboxing

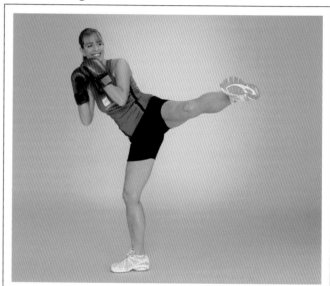

- Boxing can get your heart rate up fast, but kickboxing will keep it up longer.

- You can create more force with your lower body, so kickboxing can be a great cardio workout when done in good form and not too fast.

- There are classes, DVDs, and trainers who can help you with kickboxing. You can also shadow kickbox and do the moves without making contact.

- Start with 20 to 30 minutes of kickboxing or combine it with boxing for a total-body cardio workout.

65 percent. Take X, multiply it by .65, and then add back your RHR. This gives you the bottom of your target heart rate zone.

Let's look at an example using the formula, but keep in mind that I adjust this even a bit higher, because I still think it is too low for most people. Let's look at Sally, who is 42 years old and has a RHR of 85: 220 - 42 - 85 = 93. We multiply that by the percent she wants to use for her target heart rate zone: 93 x .65 + 85 = 145. I would probably keep Sally's low at 145 if she is in good condition .

When you become an advanced exerciser, efficiency is the most important aspect of your cardio, so you could do cardio 3 to 4 days a week for 45 to 60 minutes. But track your results and adjust as necessary.

Sprints

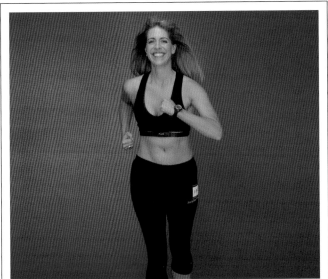

- I recommend sprints only for people who have strengthened and conditioned their bodies to handle explosive intensity on their feet, ankles, hips, and knees.

- Sprints are a good way to create an interval-training cardio session that can help burn fat more effectively.

- Keep the distance short to start. See how your body and joints feel after doing several of them.

- If you feel great, increase the number of sprints you do before increasing the distance.

Cycling

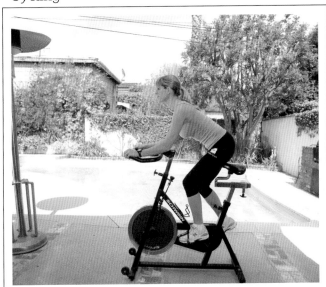

- Many people take group indoor cycling classes at every level. They love it because it is so intense.

- I have a spin bike at home that I use sometimes for cardio, because I can control how much resistance and speed I use at any given time.

- An hour-long class is an advanced form of cardio. Wear your heart rate monitor to see how your body is responding.

- I recommend a spin bike, because it can be utilized at any level.

195

ADVANCED RESISTANCE

How to use your body weight and simple tools to create more intense and advanced exercises

There are hundreds of exercises to choose for each level as you progress in your workout. The ones I chose to list here are based on my experience with people as they moved from beginner or intermediate to advanced exercises. You can do most of these exercises anywhere with little equipment, so you should put them into your toolbox of exercises.

When you reach an advanced level, you will need to increase the volume per muscle group. We will review the equation you should use to create and monitor your exercise program in the next few sections, but I want you to know that along with changing the exercises and intensity level as you progress, you will probably have to increase volume at

Stationary Lunge

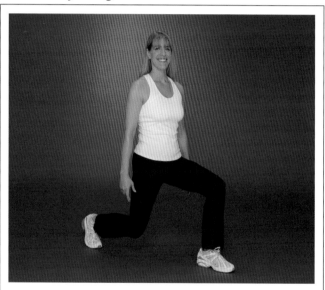

- Stand with your legs hip width apart; slide one foot behind you. Bend the front knee until it is over your ankle and then come up on your back toe to prepare for the lunge.

- Bend your back knee and lower yourself slowly toward the ground with a small range of motion. A lunge is an up-and-down motion, not forward and back.

- Start with 3 sets of 20 to 25 on each leg with no added weight.

Ball Bridge

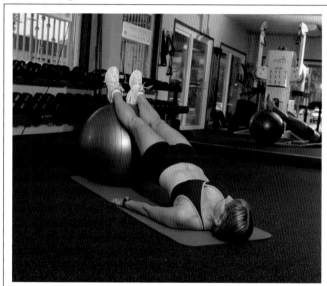

- Lie on your back and place your legs on the ball. Make sure your kneecaps are facing the ceiling.

- Push down into the ball and lift yourself up with the back of your legs. Take 2 counts to pull yourself up as high as you can go

- and then lower slowly for 2 counts.

- Do not rest on the ground in between.

- Exhale as you lift. Start with 3 sets of 30 to 35 reps.

each level as well. How much you increase it will be determined by you, your time, and your goals.

Harder exercises should still be felt mostly in your muscles, not in your joints. If you try an exercise not recommended here that you think feels extremely difficult, pay attention to where you feel it and make sure it's hard for the muscles and not for the joints.

GREEN ● LIGHT

When you get to the advanced level, try combining all three exercise suggestions from beginner to advanced. You will need more time to execute all of them, or you can divide them into body parts, but doing them all together can demonstrate how far you have progressed. You will also get a great workout that will hit most of your major muscle groups and be an intense workout for your abs! Aim to do them every 3 days.

Push-Up

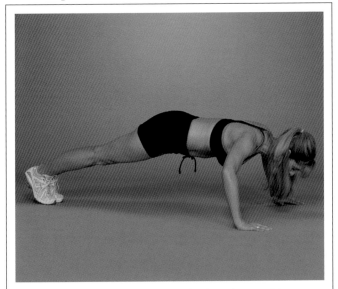

- Place your hands on the ground wider than your shoulders; your elbows should not go over your wrists when you lower yourself down.

- Your butt should be aligned with your head.

- Inhale as you lower your body; only go to 90 degrees, so your elbows are in line with your shoulders. Do not let your back dip toward the floor.

- Exhale and squeeze your abs as you push away from the ground, using 2 counts in each direction. Start with 3 sets of 10 to 15 reps.

Rear Delt Row

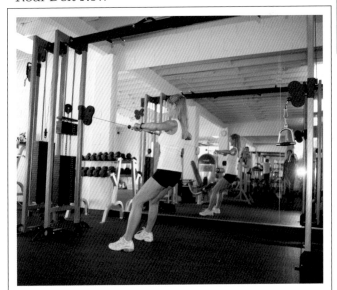

- This exercise targets the back of your shoulders, your middle back, your neck, and some biceps.

- Start with tubing at shoulder height. With palms facing down and arms extended parallel to the ground, lead with the elbows.

- Pull your arms and elbows out and back, creating a half circle on each side and then trace that line back to the start position.

- Use medium-size tubing and aim for 3 sets of 25 to 30 reps slowly with 2 counts in each direction.

DIETARY CHANGES

Making changes in your diet is critical when you commit yourself to a healthy and fit body

When you were younger, you learned to eat and like the foods that were put in front of you. And now, it's natural to gravitate toward those familiar foods that your parents fed you while you were growing up. But your taste buds can change when you decide that your health is more important than eating that fatty fried food you've been eating all your life.

Just as in exercise, making healthy food choices can be a progression. If you eat fast food several times a week, you may not be a candidate to hit the farmers' market next week or to give up fried foods tomorrow. You know yourself and your tastes well enough to make small changes that will last and can become part of your lifestyle. When you change too

Gluten Free

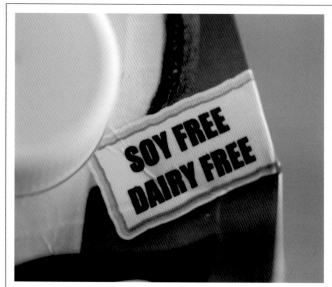

- If you have adjusted your diet to increase your results and are still stuck, I would recommend going gluten free at least temporarily.

- Gluten is inflammatory for the body, so there is no real benefit to eating anything that has it, and you can substitute most foods with a gluten-free version.

- Try it for 2 weeks and see how your body responds.

Dairy Free

- If you try going gluten free for 2 to 4 weeks and see or feel no change in your body, you might consider trying to go dairy free for 2 weeks.

- Gluten and dairy are two of the top five most common food sensitivities, so eliminating them could potentially help you to lose weight, stop the bloating and gas, and help improve your digestion.

- The more conscious you are about your health, the more willing you become to try things out.

much too soon, you don't give your body time to get used to the new flavors and change your taste or preferences.

I gave up donuts when I was in high school and have only had a bite of one since then. My tastes changed when I decided that fried dough with sugar glaze would end up as cellulite or extra body fat faster than it would do any good for me, so I quit cold turkey. I never thought I would like tofu, but I do. Progression in the diet sometimes takes longer than exercise progression, because we have such an emotional tie to foods.

If you are having trouble losing weight, it may be time to make some changes to your diet. What I hear from all my clients, and it is true for me too, is that when you eat healthier and take care of yourself and feel the difference, the stuff you wanted before becomes much less desirable.

A Shake a Day

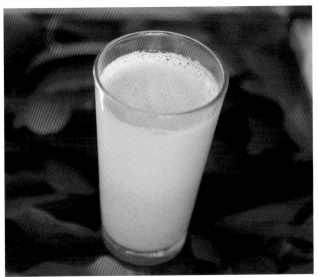

- A shake is a convenient way to get protein, vitamins, and minerals that you might not normally consume.

- Look for shakes that have at least 18 grams of protein or more per serving and make them yourself.

- There are many kinds of shakes on the market, including whey, rice, hemp, egg white, pea, and soy protein. Blend with some water, frozen berries or fruit, ground flax meal for extra fat and fiber, and anything else you want to add.

Brown Bag It

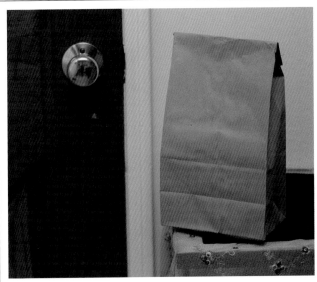

- It is much easier to stay healthy and maintain your weight when you cook your own food.

- Taking an extra 10 minutes a day to pack a healthy lunch can help you lose weight and save money.

- It might take some extra effort at first, but you can do the grocery shopping once a week and even plan a menu to make it easier and faster to prepare your lunches.

- Eating out can be fun, but it's usually much healthier to prepare your own meals.

FITT PRINCIPLE

The only equation you will ever need to create and progress in your total workout program

FITT stands for frequency, intensity, time, and type. When creating your workout program, draw two graphs and write FITT spaced out across the top of each. One graph is for cardio and the other is for resistance training. Since different exercises do different things, you want to separate them to gauge how to change or adjust them when one or both stop working. If you lump all your exercise together, then you might not be able to determine how to adjust it to get more results.

Usually people have one section that stays constant for them. For example, I worked with a woman who started an exercise program and wanted to lose over 100 pounds. When we first began, because of her fitness level, the treadmill was

Frequency

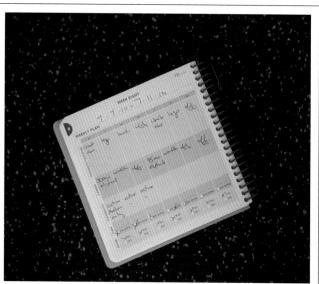

- Frequency is the number of times you commit to focused exercise each week.

- It is not the number of days necessarily, because you can do more than one workout in a day.

- Beginners might start with a frequency of 2 to 3 times

a week, while advanced exercisers aim for 4 to 5 times.

- I suggest that at least 1 day a week be a rest day with no exercise, provided that you are working hard enough when you do exercise.

Intensity

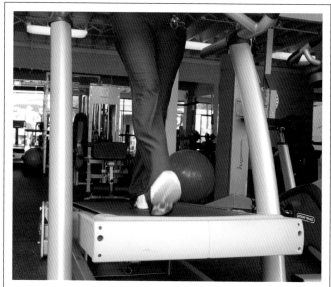

- When it comes to cardio, intensity is best judged by a heart rate monitor.

- Knowing your target heart rate zone and tracking your workouts can help you determine if the exercise you choose is the most efficient and effective for your goals.

- Using your rate of perceived exertion (RPE) is also important for both cardio and resistance training.

- A level 8 or 9 on an RPE scale for resistance training would be almost to failure.

the easiest, safest, and most effective choice for her cardio, so the type category remained the same for almost a year until she lost 80 pounds. What we adjusted along the way was the frequency, intensity, and time.

You may be someone whose biggest issue is frequency, so that column will remain the same and you might change one or more of the others over time to continue to get results. When using this equation, it is important to remember that your body is an experiment, not a math problem. What works for some may not work for you for a variety of reasons. You

track it and adjust it one step at a time to keep getting results and find what works best for you. Anytime you do the same program for months or even weeks, your body will adapt. In order to get more change, you have to adjust the environment to stimulate more change.

Time

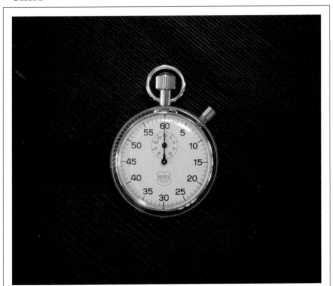

- Time is the duration of your workout. For cardio it can be from 10 or even 15 minutes to 60 or more.

- You can find benefit in 10 minutes of hard work or 30 to 40 of moderately hard work.

- When you log the time for resistance, count only the time you are exercising and then rest between each exercise.

- Start with what makes sense for you and your goals.

Type

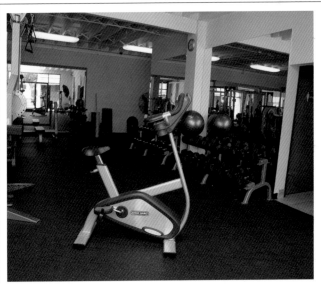

- Type is the kind of exercise you choose. Cardio examples may include walking on a treadmill, hiking, running, boxing, and swimming.

- Resistance training is the exact routine you follow, including what muscle

groups, and how many sets and reps.

- Sometimes the type you choose will be limited based on where you are and what you have access to.

- Often just changing the type can effectively produce more results.

REACHING A PLATEAU

Use the FITT principle to determine how to adjust your program so you continue to get results

I meet at least one person a week who has been doing the same workout routine for 5 years or more and wonders why he or she is not getting any more results. Luckily, after I explain the FITT principle, the client understands what he or she needs to do differently. Along your way to progressing through different levels of exercise, you will find you gravitate toward a routine that you like and do it frequently. Within the FITT principle, you may have categories like time or type that make it feel hard to make changes to your routine. This is why it really helps to have four different options for how to change your workout, and you only need to concentrate on one at a time.

Desk Job

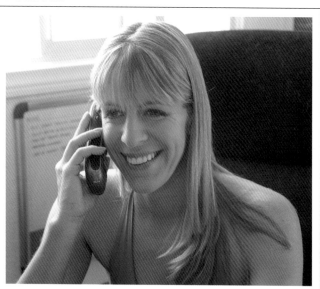

- Is your job sedentary or mobile? This is a big factor when deciding what is most important for you to concentrate on with your workouts.

- An environment change from mobile to sedentary can remove hours of low-level physical activity from your life, making it easier to gain and harder to lose weight.

- Do you get breaks in your job? Can you take the stairs instead of the elevator? Do you have your own office with a door? Look for ways to add exercise to your day if you work at a desk.

Climate

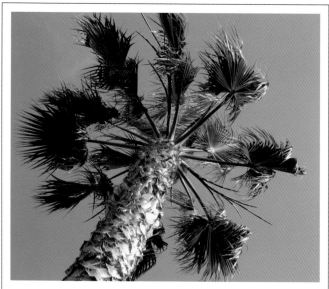

- Where you live will impact how you can work out. Do you live where it is sunny and warm or snowy and cold?

- If you live in a cold or wet climate, having indoor tools, and maybe a gym nearby, is very important to your success.

- Sunny climates increase blood levels of the hormone serotonin, so people who live in sunnier places are usually more active. If you live in a darker place, you may need extra support and tools to stay motivated.

202

Many factors go into creating a workout plan that is right for you, such as your lifestyle, goals, preferences, preexisting conditions, weather, support, and access to tools. Hopefully by now you have more tools in your workout toolbox that have become realistic options for you to replace or add into your program when your body is ready to progress to the next level. But there is no "should" about the amount of time, intensity, frequency, or type that is the gold standard. You have to decide, based on all your factors, what is most realistic and appropriate for you to add or change. When you start an exercise program that has been designed to fit everyone, it probably won't provide you with every perfect detail to fit your life and goals. You have to become your own trainer if you do not have one. Only you will be with you forever and know all the changing components in your life. Design your workout program for every aspect of your life.

Age

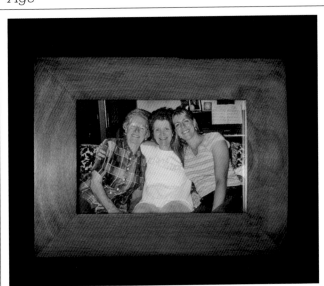

- Your age affects the choices you have for both movement and time.

- If you are in your 20s to 40s, you may be in work mode and raising a family. You may not have a lot of extra time.

- If you are over 65 and retired, you may have a ton of time. Finding exercises you love to do and that feel good are important for filling your time wisely with exercise.

- Make choices that make sense for you at every age.

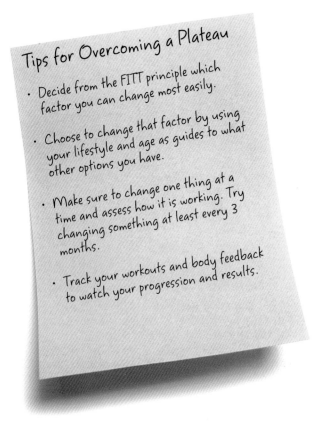

Tips for Overcoming a Plateau

- Decide from the FITT principle which factor you can change most easily.

- Choose to change that factor by using your lifestyle and age as guides to what other options you have.

- Make sure to change one thing at a time and assess how it is working. Try changing something at least every 3 months.

- Track your workouts and body feedback to watch your progression and results.

LOG YOUR PROGRESS

You have to keep track of what you do so you know when it's time to progress

It may seem tedious to you, but without a record of what you have been doing, how will you know what to change when you need to move to the next level? In fact, how will you know when it is time to move to the next level? This is why people get frustrated with exercise—they think it doesn't work because they have expectations that are not being met, when in reality they are not doing the appropriate types or volume of exercise to reach their goals.

You don't have to carry around a notebook all the time; simply log your exercise and diet once a day before you go to bed or at a meal as you are thinking about it. Unless you are in maintenance mode, you will need to do some kind of

Heart

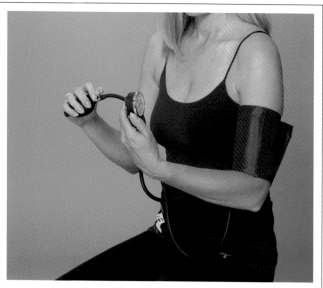

- Cardio will help you gain strength in your heart and lungs. Using a monitor or taking your pulse and tracking it can show you when you have improved.

- People often increase their aerobic capacity before seeing weight loss. Tracking

  heart rate is the first way you see the change.

- When the same level on the same machine does not increase your heart rate as much as it once did, you know you've improved.

Muscles

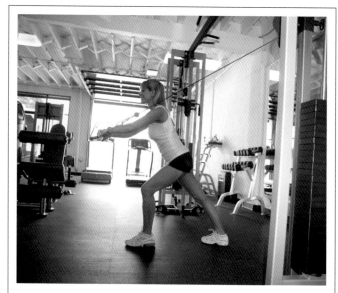

- Logging the amount of resistance you use plus the duration and frequency you exercise will help you know what to increase when your body can lift the weight easily.

- If you feel nothing at all in your body after a resistance workout, and your goal is

  to build muscle, it may be time to increase the volume or intensity.

- How you design your resistance training program can determine how you change it when you get stronger.

tracking so you know when it is time to change something about your exercise program. I like to write it down in my calendar. I use a paper calendar, but I know many people use electronic calendars. Do whatever is easiest for you. Each day I usually log my workout time, zone time, and calories from my heart rate monitor and also log what I did. This way I can go back and see how many times I needed to work out to feel at my optimum.

WHAT'S NEXT?

MAKE IT EASY

Some people track their programs on an Excel spreadsheet and do a monthly calculation of time, number of workouts, and total calories. This can provide you with a snapshot of how active you are from month to month, allowing you to see why you are getting more results one week versus the next. Aim to be efficient as well as effective.

Weight Loss

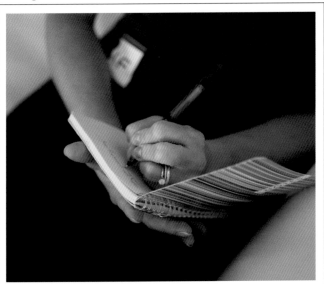

- When you begin your program, taking "before" measurements of your body fat, weight, clothing size, and waist circumference can give you some starting numbers to compare to when you want to see if your program is working.

- I would recommend remeasuring yourself no sooner than every 6 to 8 weeks for your long-term goals.

- Comparing all the numbers will offer a better picture of what kind of changes you are making rather than simply relying on the scale.

What You Eat

- People most often get stuck when it comes to their diets. Keep a food log to track what you are eating each day.

- If you are working out with intensity and frequency and still not seeing results, the obstacle may be the food.

- You can get creative about how you track your food intake—use a computer, e-mail, voicemail, PDA, or write it in a journal.

- You will not need to keep a food log forever, but you want to commit to learning about food and what to eat to best serve your body and health.

KEEP ACCOUNTABLE

Asking for support can be the difference between success and failure with your exercise program

We all have the best intentions to work out, eat healthy, and take care of ourselves. But what usually happens, as I explained in the beginning of this book, is that your exercise story and subconscious beliefs kick in to sabotage you. This is not always the case, of course. There are plenty of people who find success when they first start with exercise and

weight loss, and then they get hooked and keep it up for life. If this does not describe you, rest assured you are in the majority. Life gets in the way, and sometimes we cannot simply rely on willpower.

Aside from the tools I've already mentioned, what can you do to remain accountable? Studies show that people who

Phone Coaching

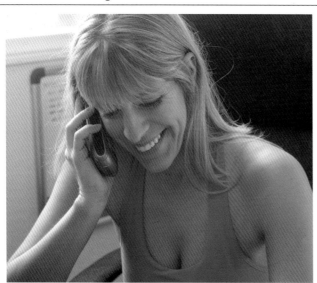

- Fitness coaching is about setting goals, creating a strategy to achieve those goals, and overcoming obstacles as they arise.

- I include fitness coaching in my programs to get people started and create better habits.

- Fitness coaching also supports you becoming independent over time and learning the skills necessary.

- You can be coached in a group or individually on exercise, weight loss, stress management, and life balance.

Internet Supervision

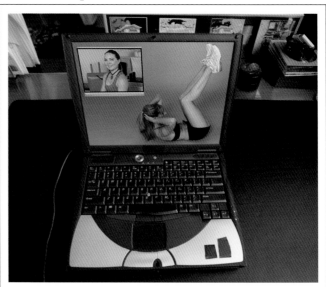

- Another way to be accountable with your workouts is to use a Web-based camera program such as Skype, which allows you to be coached as you work out.

- Some people prefer being supervised while they work out, rather than reporting back after the fact.

- Consider working with an Invisible Fitness trainer or use Skype with a trainer of your choice from all over the world.

- Today anything is possible; finding the right way to be held accountable is important for your success.

have some form of accountability do better than people who do not. Stanford University conducted a 20-year study on phone-based fitness coaching and saw adherence rates of 75 to 90 percent, which is not common in the gym. With adherence rates that high, people with a coach or a trainer experience results in fitness, strength, flexibility, and weight loss.

What if hiring someone is not possible for you right now—how can you be accountable? Start with your family or spouse, if you think he or she will support you in this process from a cheerleader perspective. You do not want to be accountable to someone you may rebel against or have emotion turmoil with. You can join a group or form a group. Gather two to ten people together once a week or on the phone to set goals and check in on results and completion from week to week. If you have tried to work out in the past and really want to commit yourself this time around, consider creating some accountability to get it done!

Forming a Support Group

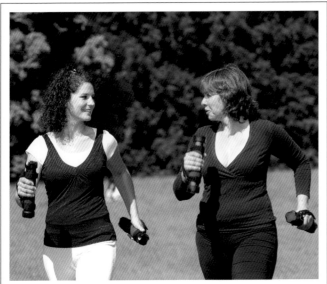

- Create a support group with like-minded people; decide what areas you want support in and how to give it to each other.

- Form a walking or hiking group that meets once a week; spend 15 to 20 minutes going over your weekly goals and accomplishments.

- Set up weekly conference calls to review your goals and accomplishments and get support along your journey. Just focus on finding like-minded people with common goals.

Logbooks

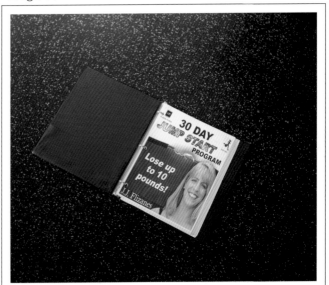

- Keeping a workout journal or logbook can help you focus on your goals, log them, and track them. Sometimes written structure is all you need to stay on track.

- You can create your own logbook; include the fields you want to track on a daily or weekly basis.

- There are programs online that you can download to track workouts, food intake, and anything else you want to be accountable for.

SHORT- & LONG-TERM GOALS

Frustration occurs when you expect too much change too soon, so set realistic goals

If you have more than 10 or 20 pounds to lose, you want to establish a series of short-term goals to keep you motivated. Over and over I see people focus on a number that they want to lose and only check in to see how close they are to that every week. Let's say you want to lose 50 pounds, so you start an exercise program. If you do it safely and change

your lifestyle as you go, it may take you a year or more to accomplish your goal. There are fast weight-loss programs out there, but they are not all healthy, and most people fail at them because they do not adjust their lifestyles at the same time.

Imagine that you're 2 weeks into your program and have

Try on Clothing

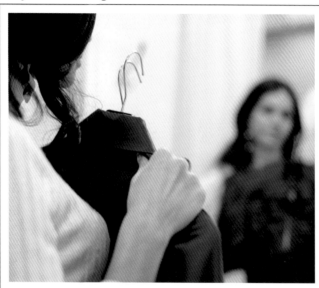

- Start with some clothes that you can almost fit into. Make it a short-term goal that you will get into a pair of tighter jeans in 2 to 3 months.

- Create your plan and then try them on at the end of 8 weeks to see where you are.

- If you carry your weight up top, choose a shirt that is snug.

- Hide the clothing in the back of your closet, but mark on your calendar when it is time to pull them out.

Measure Inches

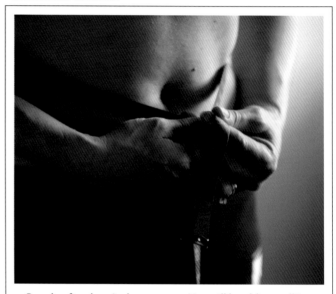

- People often lose inches before they lose weight. Taking your measurements can show you that you are on the right track.

- Even if your weight is the same, you may have lost some body fat or inches off your waist and gained muscle.

- You will be able to tell in your clothes, but you might not be able to quantify the changes.

- Take measurements from both sides of your body from head to toe.

been extremely disciplined about your diet and exercise. You have more energy, and you feel your body slowly changing. One morning you step on the scale, expecting it to show results—but you see no change. This happens to a lot of us. For some reason people put on weight and remain sedentary for years, but then expect major changes just a few short weeks into their program. Do you understand how expectations like this can undermine your entire weight-loss plan? It did not take you 2 weeks to put on weight, so it's going to take a lot longer to get it off. Remember, too: If you do not change your thoughts, feelings, habits, and lifestyle along with diet and exercise, any weight loss will be temporary.

What are some short-terms goals you could set to keep you motivated along your journey? I have listed some below, but get creative and add more that better fit your life. Keep your eye on the long-term but acknowledge yourself every step of the way.

Run or Walk a 5K

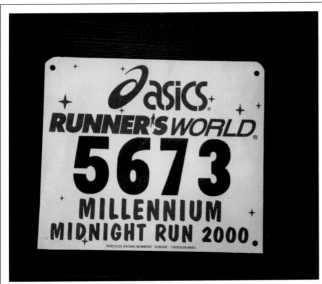

- A lot of my clients want accountability with a goal for their cardio; I usually suggest a 5K to start.

- A 5K is 5 kilometers, or 3.1 miles. You can usually find one being held in your area.

- Training for an event gives you a deadline, so it can keep you motivated and disciplined.

- It doesn't have to be a running race—it could be biking, hiking or walking. Find an event that you would be excited to do.

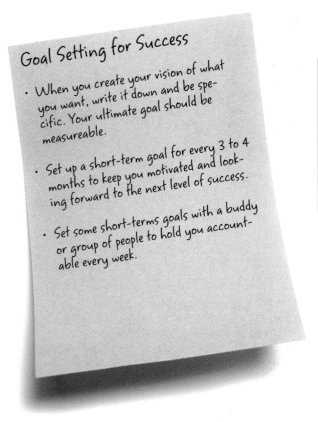

Goal Setting for Success

- When you create your vision of what you want, write it down and be specific. Your ultimate goal should be measureable.

- Set up a short-term goal for every 3 to 4 months to keep you motivated and looking forward to the next level of success.

- Set some short-terms goals with a buddy or group of people to hold you accountable every week.

REWARDS

Implementing a reward structure to keep you motivated can also help get you results

If working out feels like work to you, then maybe try a reward for yourself to keep you motivated and inspired. I love to work out and take care of myself, but I also like to take time to acknowledge the hard work and dedication I have given to my work and health. The list of rewards on these pages represents only a few items from a long list of things from which you can choose. You do not have to spend a lot of—or even any—money; just be sure to reward yourself with things that you truly enjoy. Taking time to reward yourself and savor your accomplishments can actually help you get results, because rewards can help you manage your stress and hormones. Make rewarding yourself a part of your plan;

Massage

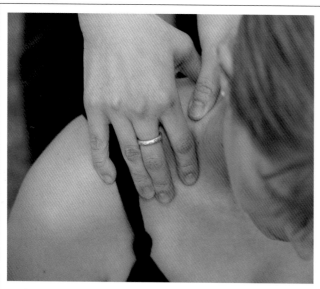

- There are massage places available for every budget. From the chair massage at the mall for ten bucks to the five-star spa massage for several hundred.

- If someone in your life likes to give massages, make them a meal in exchange for a free massage.

- Some people prefer a facial or reflexology over a massage—the point is simply to pamper yourself.

- Massage will help with lymph drainage and hormone and energy levels, so it can actually help you with your goals.

Pedicure

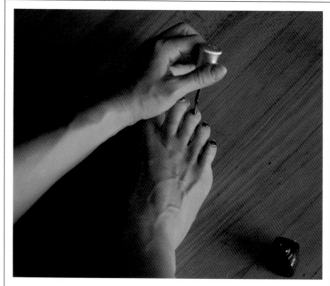

- Whether you get polish or not, a pedicure is a time to take care of your feet, which are the foundation of a lot of your workouts.

- When feet hurt, people do not work out as much. Taking care of your feet is important for the longevity of your foundation.

- Have one alone or make it a party with some friends and snacks. Get some girl and pamper time!

place it in the stress-management and fun category. When you focus on fun and rewards, you stop worrying so much about the results—and that can also help balance your mind and body.

We live in a fast-paced, stress-filled time, and we have the option to ride the wave of fear about something or decide to turn our attention to what is working and what is going well. That translates to the way you treat yourself and your body.

Shopping

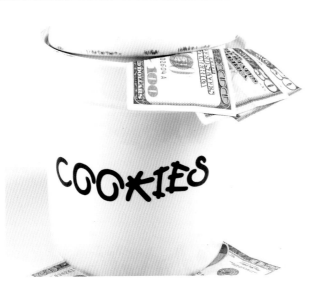

- If you are saving up for that special outfit, why not make it a reward for achieving your goals?

- For every week you accomplish your goal, put a certain amount of money aside to spend on that special outfit.

- You could choose something that does not fit you perfectly yet; make it a goal to get into it.

- You can also choose a piece of jewelry or furniture—whatever gets you excited and motivated.

Dinner Out

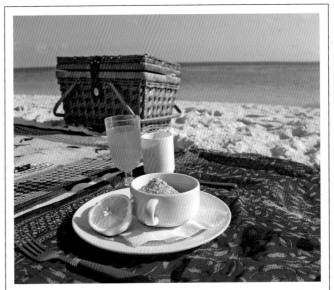

- Plan and save for a special dinner out at your favorite restaurant.

- It does not have to be expensive, but it should be special enough that it gets you excited and keeps you motivated.

- A dinner cruise, a picnic on the beach, a home-cooked meal by your family—these are all options.

- Try not to focus on the food as the reward but the experience and company you keep. Food should be enjoyed, but the main event should be whom you are with and where you are.

211

BREAKFAST SUGGESTIONS

Start your day off right with some substantial protein for lasting energy and focus

The biggest problem with the typical American breakfast is that it contains too much sugar and simple carbohydrates. From previous chapters, I am sure you're not surprised that I recommend limiting carbohydrates to mostly vegetables and fruits and increasing protein intake.

We wonder why kids cannot concentrate in school when we give them sugar in the form of sweet cereal before they head out the door. When you eat a simple carbohydrate for breakfast, it will be digested and broken down quickly. This will lead to a potential spike in your blood sugar and then an empty gas tank. This is why people get hungry 2 hours after eating cereal or a simple carbohydrate for breakfast.

Eggs

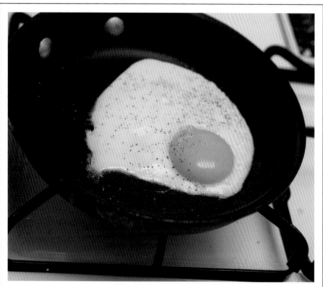

- Eggs are so versatile that you can prepare them in many ways before becoming bored.

- Try eggs over easy, scrambled, poached, hard-boiled, sunny-side up, deviled, or in a salad, omelet, or quiche.

- You can add all kinds of vegetables to an omelet, or you can sauté some veggies to have as a side dish with eggs.

- Two eggs are around 140 calories and have about 14 grams of protein. And egg white has 15 to 20 calories and 4.7 grams of protein.

Protein Shake

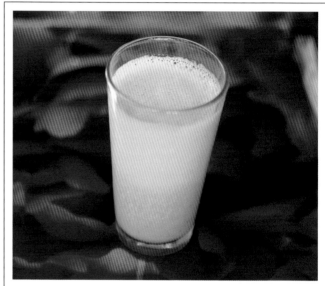

- A shake is a great meal replacement for breakfast, because you can pack it with good nutrients.

- Whey is one of the most common proteins but other choices include egg white, hemp, pea, and rice protein.

- Use a 1/2 cup frozen berries or other fruit, add a spoonful of your favorite nut butter for fat, and some cinnamon or vanilla for flavor.

- Use water and add ice to thicken. You can add some extra fiber, probiotics, and greens for an extra healthy shake.

For every meal we need to focus on the protein source and the fruits and veggies first. Then we want some healthy fat added to help slow down absorption of these nutrients and to help us feel full longer. The recommendations on these pages have many variations and ways to prepare them.

Some of your favorite foods may come in a healthier form, so make sure to read food labels and do a little homework. Spending a little extra money for good quality that keeps your body healthy is a better investment than skimping and being cheap, only to pay for it later in doctor bills.

Steel-Cut Oatmeal

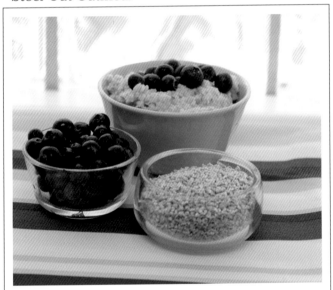

- Steel-cut oatmeal has more protein and fiber than quick or rolled oats.

- This type of oatmeal takes longer to cook, but you can have leftovers throughout the week.

- Try adding dried apricots, slivered almonds, and cinnamon for extra fiber, healthy fat, and the anti-inflammatory benefits of cinnamon.

- You can also add 1/4 to 1/2 cup to Greek yogurt for some extra protein. I like mine with a touch of honey, too.

Breakfast Sausage

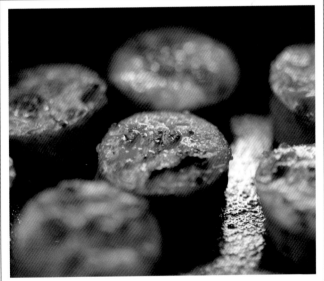

- There are many kinds of sausage: chicken, turkey, beef, and veggie. Look for a link with a protein content of 18 to 22 grams as a substantial breakfast.

- You can replace sausage links with a patty. Try grilling chicken patties in the morning as well.

- If you are a vegan or vegetarian, you can stir-fry some tempeh with onions. Tempeh is a great protein choice; it also helps with digestion, because it is a fermented food that contains probiotics.

JJ'S FAVORITE SHAKE

Protein powders are not created equal in nutrition or taste

For convenience's sake, I make a shake at least once a day to replace one of my meals, so I have tried many different variations to find the few combinations I like. Because everyone has different taste, you should experiment with many kinds and flavors to find one you like best. Before I did my food-sensitivity test, I enjoyed vanilla and chocolate whey protein. Because it is made from milk, whey has a creamy taste to it that makes you think it could be a milkshake! When I decided

to try following a dairy-free diet for a few months, I had to explore the other type of proteins out there. Egg white protein is my next favorite followed by a specific brand of hemp protein. Each shake needs adjustments to make the best flavor. When using hemp protein, you may want to add a banana to cut the "green" taste a bit and to add some natural sweetness.

Step one is to find the kind of protein you like: whey, hemp,

Picking Protein

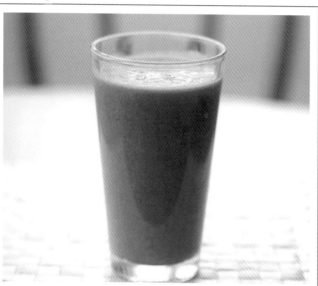

- When choosing a powder, look for one that has at least 10 to 15 grams of protein per scoop.

- Read the label to know if you need one scoop or two per shake. Start with water in the blender first and then add the powder so it does

not get stuck to the bottom of the blender.

- Using water keeps the calories down and gives you more water in your diet. Milks and juices will increase calories and sugar quickly, so dilute them if you feel you need to use them.

Adding Extra Sweetness

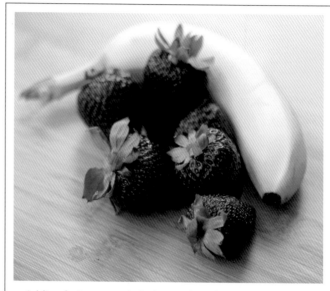

- Adding fruit to your shake is a better choice than adding juice. The fruit gives you less sugar and more fiber and it can make the shake thicker.

- If you use fresh fruit, add an ice cube or two to chill the shake and make it thick. You can also use frozen fruit.

- Strawberries and bananas are the most common fruit to use in shakes, because they are easy to find and add natural sugar.

egg white, brown rice. Step two is to add some fresh or frozen fruit with some water as a base. Step three is to add any extra flavorings and a little healthy fat to make the shake a satisfying meal replacement.

Choosing Fruit

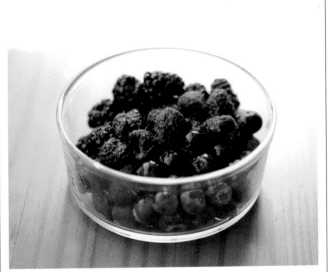

- Berries are a great way to get more antioxidants in your diet.

- Raspberries are high in fiber, and blueberries contain more antioxidants than almost any other fruit.

- Start by using one or two of your favorites fruits in your shake. Be sure to try different combinations to find your favorite.

- Use 1/4 to 1/2 cup fruit to start. Taste as you go in case you want to add or change something; write down any combinations you create that you really love!

Choosing Fat, Fiber, and Flavor

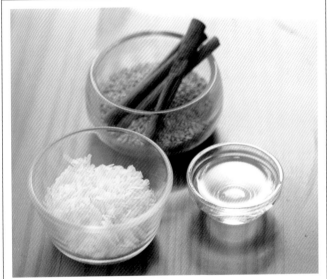

- To make your shake a complete meal that will satiate you for 4 to 5 hours, you need to add some healthy fat.

- Flaxseeds, coconut flakes, and nut butters are the three most common fats that I use.

- Add 1 tablespoon of your favorite fat to start. You can also choose coconut cream, ground nuts, or toasted flaxseeds; these will give your shake a nutty flavor.

LUNCH OPTIONS

Get creative with salads that you can eat at home, at work, or on the run

The tuna, chicken, and egg salads described on these pages are versatile and can serve as a snack as well as a meal. You can have them on a slice of gluten-free bread for an open-faced sandwich, or you can scoop some onto a bed of greens for a salad (use the creaminess of the mayonnaise as the dressing). For a special treat add a slice of cheese or shredded non-dairy cheese to the open-faced chicken or tuna salad sandwich and toast it for a special lunch. You can also eat these salads with celery sticks or crackers for an easily transportable lunch. Having options for lunch on the go is important to me, as I spend most of my time training clients, teaching classes, and lecturing.

Tuna Salad

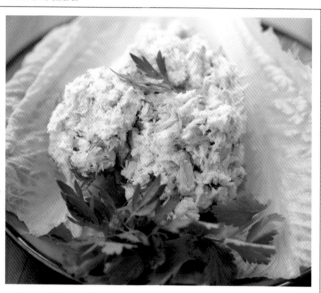

- Start with your favorite can or pouch of tuna. I use three cans to make tuna salad for the week.

- Make sure to drain it completely, and even consider rinsing it if you are watching your sodium.

- For three cans of tuna, I use 1/2 to 3/4 cup mayo, but I usually use a spoon and add what I need to get the texture I like.

- Using a fork, mix up the mayo and tuna until it is as creamy as you like it.

Chicken Salad

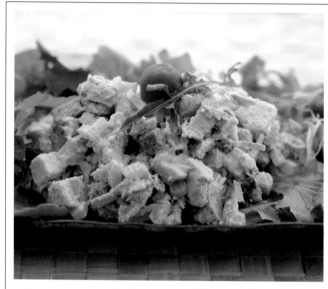

- Since the chicken for this dish is combined with other flavors, I often use plain grilled chicken.

- You can also use canned chicken or rotisserie if you do not have a grill, but fresh is best.

- Cube the grilled chicken or shred it, depending on how you are going to serve it and how you like it.

- Add mayo, mustard, and spices to taste. Fresh herbs, Italian dressing, garlic, and onion are nice ways to spice up chicken salad.

These options provide protein and fat as well as carbohydrates and fiber when you add vegetables or eat them on top of a bed of greens. How much fat and protein you get will depend on how you make each salad. The more mayo you use, the more fat and calories there will be. You can substitute some of the mayo with Italian dressing and mustard to shave off some fat and calories.

Remember that eating fat does not mean you gain more fat, so I would prefer you eat a little more mayo and a lot less starchy carbs like bread and crackers. There are also vegan mayonnaise options available. Every different kind of mayo will change the taste, so be sure to test them out before using them in a big batch of salad. You can also create your own salad using pork, turkey, salmon, or whitefish.

Egg Salad

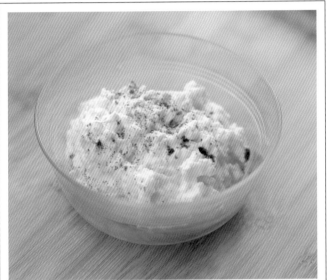

- Start by hard-boiling some eggs and letting them cool off before peeling and separating.

- I like to use one egg yolk for every three egg whites, because I prefer the taste and want the fat to come from the mayo instead of the yolk.

- Unless you have cholesterol levels in the danger zones, eat egg yolks if you like them.

- I separate the cooled whites and yolks, cut the whites up very small, and then add the yolks in a mash together with the mayo.

Spice It Up

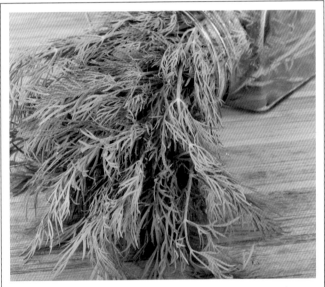

- Growing and using fresh herbs such as dill, fennel, cilantro, and parsley can help add a burst of flavor to a common dish.

- Fresh herbs have fuller flavor compared to dried herbs. Try adding a pinch of freshly ground pepper!

- Adding Dijon mustard or spicy brown mustard can also kick up the flavor in any of these salads.

- Chopped celery, green onions, nuts, or even apples can enhance the tuna and chicken salads, while paprika can kick-start egg salad.

JJ'S HOMEMADE VEGETABLE SOUP

Get your daily dose of green leafy vegetables in a delicious homemade soup

Do you eat at least four to six servings of vegetables every day? Most of us do not. With a busy lifestyle, sometimes I find it takes more effort to get in green leafy vegetables on a daily basis. A few years ago I decided to start making vegetable soup in order to get my daily recommended servings of vegetables and to have something green in my diet every day.

With soup you can add all the ingredients that you like and try different combinations. If you do not like green vegetables, this is a great way to have them with some spices that make them more interesting and tasty. I used to buy kale, Swiss chard, and zucchini with the hopes that I would eat them fresh regularly, but they would wind up going bad in

Ingredients

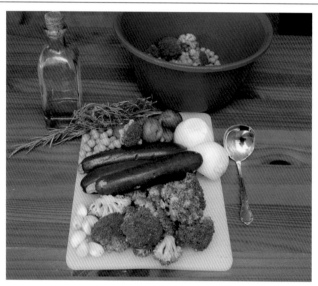

- For this soup I use zucchini, yellow squash, onions, garlic, broccoli, a few small red potatoes, and some chickpeas for protein.

- You can also add cashews for some protein and fat. They make soup creamy.

- I have also made soups with dark green leafy vegetables like kale, spinach, Swiss chard, and collard greens.

- The potatoes and chickpeas give the soup a thicker consistency at the end when it's blended all together.

Cutting the Veggies

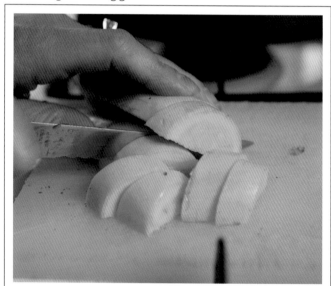

- Since the veggies are cooked and then blended, you can cut them in medium to large slices.

- If you do not want to puree the soup at the end, then cut small pieces; be sure to chop the onion and garlic into small pieces.

- I usually start with some olive oil in a big pot and sauté the onions and garlic for a few minutes.

- I start with a few tablespoons of olive oil and add more if necessary, depending on the amount of veggies I use.

my refrigerator before I could eat them all because of my schedule.

Making a soup is easy, and reheating it is even easier! Make sure you have a large soup jar or container and have room in your refrigerator to store it. I would recommend making this soup once a week or every 2 weeks and consuming it within 7 days. You can also freeze it to enjoy later.

I add beans or nuts to the soup for some added fat and protein, but you can also add protein after the soup has been blended together. Chicken, pork, beef, tofu, or tempeh can make this a complete meal. You can also top it off with some cheese or tortilla strips to add some extra flavor for a dinner or side dish. Another fun combination is carrot, beet, and ginger. The color of your soup will depend upon the vegetables you use and the quantity you add.

Cooking It All Together

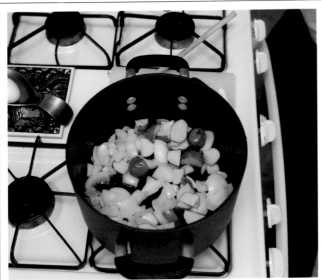

- After the onions and garlic are cooked a little, add the potatoes and any harder vegetables in next; these need to cook longer.

- Continue to chop and add vegetables into the pot.

- Add some garlic powder, a little high-mineral salt, and freshly ground pepper and other spices, such as cilantro, dill, or oregano to taste.

- Fill the pot with water and any broth to flavor it. I use 1 to 2 cups chicken broth with water, or I just use water.

The Finished Product

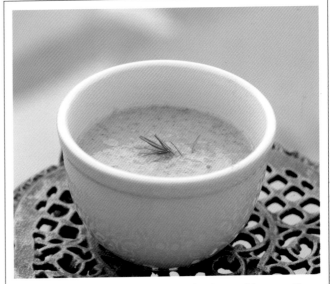

- Bring the mixture to a boil; simmer on medium heat for 30 to 45 minutes, until veggies are very soft.

- Turn off the burner and let the pot of veggies cool down for at least 30 minutes.

- Blend everything together either in a blender or food processor and add any additional salt, pepper, and spices to taste.

- Enjoy your first fresh bowl or share it with family and let the rest cool off before storing.

HEALTHY DINNERS
Using your grill can make dinner easy, healthy, fun, and fast

When you have time to cook, being creative and preparing meals can be a rewarding experience. Personally, I love to cook. But when life gets busy, people too often resort to fast food or unhealthy choices. I understand what it is like to be busy, so I have chosen meals to share with you based on what I do myself on a regular basis, when I have little time to be extra creative in the kitchen. When it comes to dinner, grilling is one of the easiest, healthiest, and fastest options.

There are indoor and outdoor grills—and even stovetop grills for people who have a small kitchen space to work with. Panfrying and baking normally mean added fat and calories from oil. A grill can give a smoked flavor naturally without added fats.

Marinate the meats and fish in the spices of your choice either overnight or for a few hours. This will save you time and add more flavor to your meal. I have centered my

Salmon and Asparagus

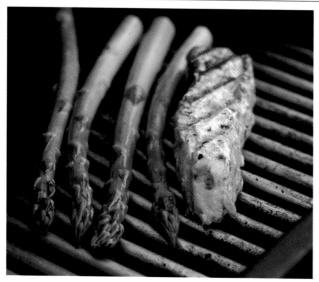

- Wild salmon is filled with healthy, antiaging omega-3 fatty acids and has a full flavor.

- You can grill, poach, panfry, or bake it—or have it smoked.

- Asparagus is also great on the grill, either cooked on an open flame or in foil with some olive oil, salt, and pepper. You can also roast it on a cookie sheet in a 400°F oven for 10 minutes.

- You can add some soy sauce or lemon to this simple dish.

Beef and Broccoli

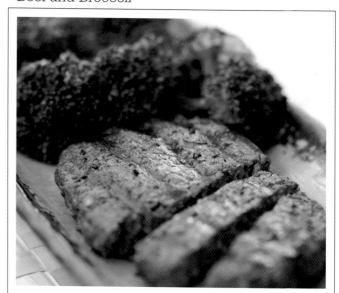

- There are many kinds of red meat you can use, like buffalo, tri-tip, ground beef, sirloin, and other kinds of steak.

- An average portion size would be 2 to 5 ounces, depending on the person. Make sure to get lean cuts that are organic.

- I use a steamer to steam the broccoli while the beef is cooking on the grill. Add some spices or sauces for more taste if you desire.

recommendations on a protein and vegetable choice. You can also add sauces or fresh herbs to taste to all the meal suggestions. Aim for 2 to 5 ounces of protein and at least 2 cups of veggies at dinner.

YELLOW ●LIGHT

If you need to add another carbohydrate, choose a gluten-free option like rice, potatoes, or quinoa to accompany your meal. But when you can, add more vegetables before adding starches at dinner, because the body usually slows down at night and does not need the same amount of calories as it might in the middle of the day, when it needs more energy.

Grilled Chicken Salad

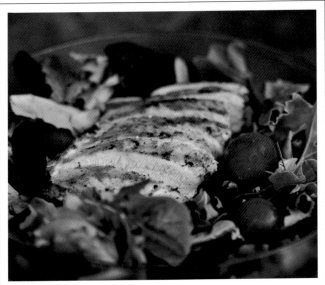

- Having a salad for dinner is a great way to watch your calories and prepare your body for sleep.

- You can cut up a simple grilled chicken breast and toss it into a bed of greens.

- Chop some cucumber, tomatoes, and any other salad veggies you like and add your favorite dressing.

- I love to add extra flavor to my salads with some feta cheese, avocado, sesame seeds, cranberries, or walnuts.

Ahi Tuna and Spinach

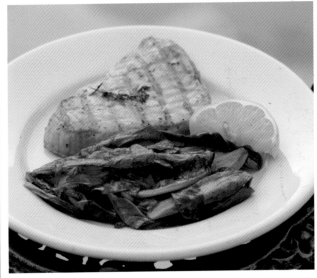

- Tuna is high in omega-3 fatty acids and can help lower cholesterol.

- If you do not eat raw fish, you may want to cook it through instead of searing it. In that case, you will need to add some fat to moisten it.

- Sauté spinach in olive oil with a touch of garlic powder and pepper. Spinach cooks down fast; don't be shy and fill the pan to start.

- I use a gluten-free soy sauce with this dish to add more flavor to the tuna.

GUILTLESS DESSERTS
Save room for some tasty treats that are actually good for you

If you want another reason to eliminate the starchy carbs at dinner, it's dessert. I love dessert, so to me, it's worth it to eat a little less at dinner to save room for these treats. If you have a sweet tooth or just enjoy having something to clean your palate after dinner, you can choose something that not only tastes good but actually has nutritional value too. Replace that cake, pie, or muffin with one of these suggestions. Aside from the angel food cake, everything else is also gluten free.

If you do not have a sweet tooth, be grateful and skip the dessert and enjoy some wine! Red wine has antioxidants, and champagne has been found to be good for your brain (in moderation, of course), so have a glass as your dessert instead. If you are out at a restaurant, share a dessert with two or three people. This is a great way to get a taste of something you love without eating the entire portion. You will have had a treat and saved some money at the same time.

Coconut Ice Cream

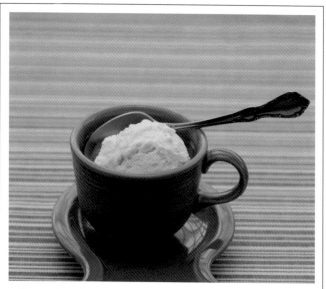

- Remember: Coconut is good for you. Since trying a dairy-free lifestyle, I have been introduced to coconut ice cream.

- It comes in many flavors, so you are not limited to one, and you can do all the same things with it as you would regular ice cream.

- A scoop or two with some fruit makes a perfect dessert on a hot, summer day.

- Make a shake or sundae with it, or serve it to the kids in cones. They may not notice the difference.

Dark Chocolate

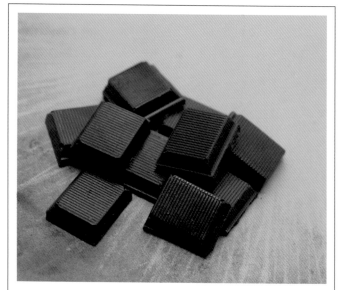

- Dark chocolate is very high in antioxidants and is gluten free.

- You won't need much but a bite or two to satisfy a sweet tooth after dinner. Break out a bar and share it around the table, or break off a piece or two for you and store the rest.

- The higher the cocoa, the more bitter it is. If you are making the transition from milk to dark, start with less cocoa and work your way up as your palate adjusts.

A great way to choose a dessert is to know its nutritional value. Sugar by itself will spike blood sugar at any meal, so look for items that have protein, fat, and/or fiber. Choose your dessert to complement your dinner. If you have a heavier dinner, choose berries or fruit for dessert. If you have a salad or something light for dinner, enjoy a piece of angel food cake or some gluten-free cookies for dessert. Try to plan ahead to make the best choices for all your meals throughout your day. Successful weight management entails looking at the whole picture and working backward sometimes.

Berries

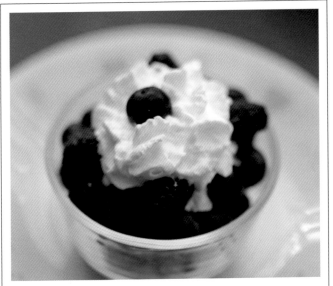

- Berries with whipped cream or yogurt are a refreshing treat after dinner; they provide antioxidants and some fiber disguised as dessert.

- Whipped cream can transform berries into a treat, and if you are dairy free try rice whip or soy whip.

- Top them off with some coconut flakes or almond slices for extra flavor.

- Mix them in some Greek yogurt with honey for added protein.

Angel Food Cake

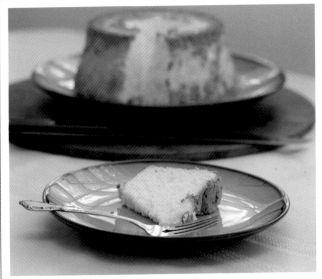

- If you want a cake, why not choose one with protein in it?

- Angel food cake is made mostly of egg whites.

- You can add some berries, whipped cream, or even coconut ice cream if you want to spice it up.

- If you make it yourself, you can choose to use gluten-free flour, and then it's a very healthy cake choice for dessert.

GLUTEN-FREE DECADENT COOKIES

Redesign your favorite recipes so you can still enjoy your favorite treats

When I decided to try a dairy-free and chocolate-free diet for a few months to help strengthen my immune and digestive systems, I needed to find or create a treat I could have after dinner. Dairy and chocolate were two of my favorite foods but I knew my cravings were telling me that my body was not able to digest them properly. Giving them up was challenging because no one likes restrictions, but most people love replacements! I took an already gluten-free cookie recipe and changed the ingredients. The original cookie was a peanut butter and chocolate chip cookie, which I turned into a sunflower butter, vegan carob chip cookie. Not the same, but good enough!

Carob Chip Cookies

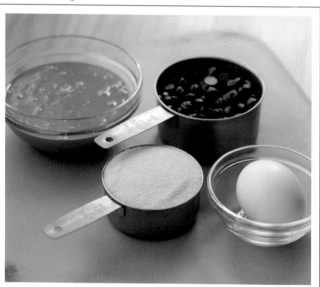

- In a bowl, combine 1 cup nut butter (peanut, almond, or sunflower), 1 cup chocolate or carob chips, 1/2 to 1/3 cup sugar, and 1 egg.

- If you use sunflower butter, you can add 1/4 to 1/2 cup gluten-free flour to make the batter less sticky.

- You can use vegan carob chips, chocolate chips, or any kinds of chips you like.

- The original recipe calls for 1 cup sugar, which I found to be too much, so I have reduced it to 1/2 to 1/3.

Mixing Together

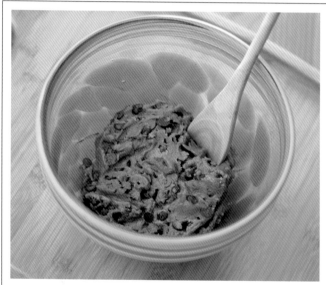

- Beat the egg first and then add the nut butter and sugar.

- If you are going to add some flour, add it before adding the chips.

- Add the chips last and mix the batter all together. The batter is sticky because it's mostly nut butter.

- You can freeze or refrigerate the batter in case you are not ready to put the cookies on a baking sheet.

If you love something, giving it up is hard. If you can replace it with something healthier that your body can digest better, then you will be both physically and emotionally more satisfied. Plus, trying new foods can help you discover new favorites that you might not have tried before. My new favorite "treat" is sunflower butter. I love it! And I never would have tried it if I wasn't experimenting with new foods. You can redesign any recipe you love and adjust it to make it healthier.

On the Cookie Sheet

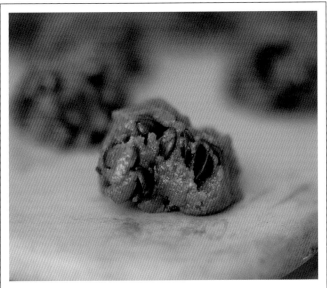

- I use two spoons to scoop the batter and form it into a ball-like shape on the cookie sheet.

- Preheat the oven to 350°F and make sure to leave enough room on the cookie sheet for them to expand.

- If you did not use flour, the cookies will expand.

- If you used flour, you will want to use a fork to flatten them out toward the end of the baking time.

Finished Cookies

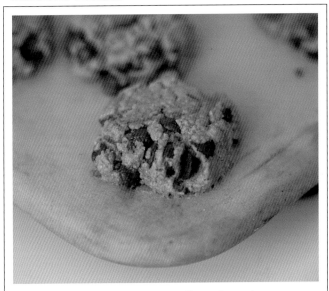

- Bake for 10 to 12 minutes, and let the cookies cool 5 or 10 minutes before removing them from the cookie sheet.

- Enjoy the cookies warm or cold. I let them cool off and then store them in an airtight container to enjoy over time.

- The recipe makes over a dozen, depending on how much batter you use for each cookie.

- Get creative with the recipe. Try honey instead of sugar, add some vanilla or cinnamon, and experiment with different nut butters.

RECOMMENDED SNACKS

Eat a snack that has some protein and fiber to help maintain your blood sugar level

If you are always on the go, having a few staple snacks is important to staying on track with your diet and health. Eating every 4 to 5 hours will keep your blood sugar and energy levels high; you will feel good and alert throughout your day. If you think you could be without food for more than 5 hours, you should have some snacks ready to go to prevent you from crashing. Remember that your body uses muscles for energy when your gas tank is on empty; meal planning and snacks are crucial to maintain your metabolism and achieve successful weight management.

I chose the snacks on these pages because this is what I eat with my on-the-go busy lifestyle. You can replace these with

Fruit and Nuts

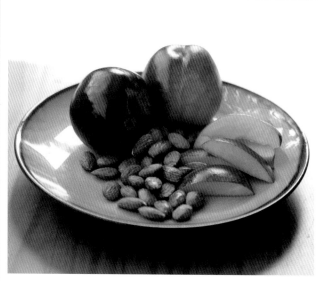

- I keep nuts in my car at all times for when I get hungry on the go.

- Nuts have fat and protein and store easily. A quarter cup is approximately 170 calories and is usually enough to satisfy a craving.

- Nectarines, peaches, plums, and apples are easy to take on the go because you do not need to peel them. Do not leave them in your car.

- Dried fruit in moderation can be a perfect choice when you want something sweet. Control portions and sugar content.

Jerky

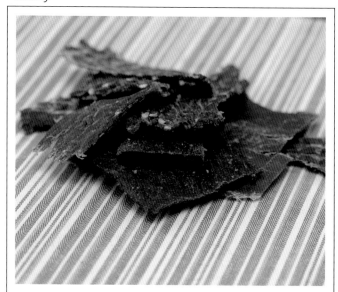

- In writing this book, I actually discovered a few types of jerky that I did not know existed!

- There is beef jerky, turkey jerky, ahi tuna jerky, and tofurkey jerky. These are not a good choice if you are watching your sodium.

- Like meat in general, find a jerky that is raised without antibiotics and is organic and gluten free.

- Jerky has a lot of protein and a long shelf life, so you can store it in your car as an emergency snack.

a dinner or lunch choice when you have time to prepare and cook. But I know that most people who do not think ahead let themselves suffer when they are hungry. They wind up eating some processed, fast-food item that ultimately will not help their overall goal of weight loss and healthy living. I have a plastic shoebox with a lid in my car that I fill with healthy snacks so I am never without a good choice.

············ GREEN ● LIGHT ············

Make sure to pack your car, backpack, purse, or briefcase with at least two healthy snacks in case you miss a meal or get caught in between meals. The items here do not spoil as rapidly as some others, so make sure to keep in mind the conditions of your car or purse when choosing what snacks to pack. Also make sure to always carry water with you as well.

Canned Sardines or Oysters

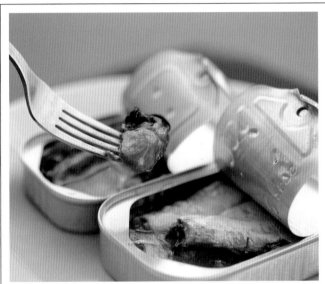

- I love canned sardines and oysters because they are usually canned in olive oil and do not need to be refrigerated.

- They are high in protein and omega-3 fatty acids. They also travel easily, which is great if you are always on the go.

- I eat oysters with gluten-free crackers or tortilla chips and eat the sardines right out of the can.

- You can also throw them on a salad. I know they are an acquired taste, but try them!

Protein Bar

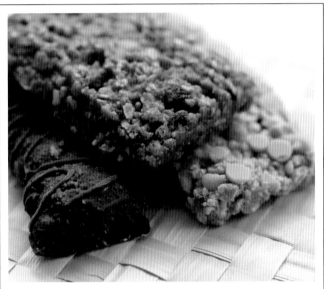

- There are many bars on the market; choosing one can be tricky.

- Make sure to read labels and see how much protein and sugar are in the bars you choose.

- If eaten as a meal replacement, you need well over 15 grams of protein. But if you have it as a snack, aim for 5 to 10.

- Make sure you know all or most of the ingredients in the bars you eat. Avoid those that have too many preservatives and chemicals.

5-STEP FITNESS PLAN

Step #1: Create a Vision

Write out your goals very specifically, and journal about the picture in your mind that you want to create. Post some goals where you can see them. Take some measurements and body fat percentage and then put the scale away for three months! Keep your journal handy to log your progress, how you are feeling, and what you are doing each week. Use these Resources pages to get you started.

What are your fitness goals?

_____

_____

_____

What clear picture can you create?

_____

_____

_____

What are the ways you will know you have gotten results?

_____

_____

_____

Step #2: Make a Plan

Aim for one small goal every week and one larger goal every mo Get a grocery list ready of the things you want to stock up on to h you be successful.

Do you have a step by step plan? Explain.

_____

_____

_____

Do you have alternative routes? Explain.

_____

_____

_____

Is your plan tailored for you in all areas? Explain.

_____

_____

_____

Do you have cardio and resistance training in your plan? Explain.

_____

_____

_____

How will you stick to it each week?

_____

_____

_____

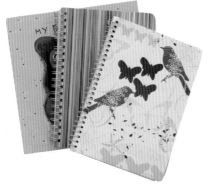

228

Step #3: Progression

Use the FITT principle to help you chart your progress. When the program is comfortable and easy, it might not be enough.

Are you tracking your progress? Explain.

_____

_____

_____

When you stop seeing results and it is time to adjust your program, what is your next step?

_____

_____

_____

What are you going to change to get to the next level?

_____

_____

_____

Step #4: Tools and Support

What tools are you using now?

_____

_____

_____

What tools should you be using?

_____

_____

_____

Have you set up a support foundation around you to support your goals?

_____

_____

_____

Do you have support for both your mind and body?

_____

_____

_____

If you lack support, how do you deal with that?

_____

_____

_____

Step #5: Joint Integrity

Do you have any joint injuries? If so, list.

_____

_____

_____

Do you choose exercises to protect your joints? If so, list.

_____

_____

_____

Is your joint health important to you? Explain.

_____

_____

_____

PERSONALIZING YOUR FITNESS PLAN

Creating Your Vision

Describe in detail who you want to be when it comes to your fitness, health, and body. List every aspect that is important to you as it pertains to every area of your life.

_____

_____

_____

_____

_____

_____

Why is this vision and goal important to you?

_____

_____

_____

_____

_____

What obstacles get in the way of getting here?

_____

_____

_____

_____

_____

What are your strengths that will help you overcome these obstac

_____

_____

_____

_____

_____

What is one action you can take today toward this goal that you not currently doing?

_____

_____

_____

_____

_____

Measuring Yourself

I would HIGHLY recommend doing this so you may see what changes you have made after 60 or 90 days of your new program. However, I do not want you to weigh yourself every day or even every week. Numbers can help us see changes we otherwise may not notice, but they can also be the source of confusion and frustration if you allow it. Have someone else help you with this so you can get an accurate reading at the end. I also recommend that the SAME person help you at the end with the same materials to measure you. Treat this as a scientific experiment and do everything as identical as you can—from the time of day to the clothes you are wearing. Use a mirror to make sure your measuring tape is straight. After you weigh in, put the scale away for at least 60 days.

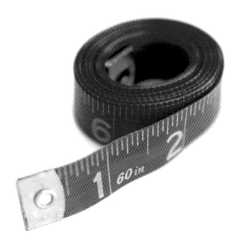

Date: _____

Height: _____

Present Weight: _____

Body Fat %: _____
(Use website on page 234.)

Measurements
Use a standard tape measure

Measure from elbow to shoulder and record the measurement in the middle

Upper Arm Left: _____

Upper Arm Right: _____

Measure at nipple line

Chest: _____

Measure around body

Waist at navel: _____

Waist at smallest: _____

Measure with feet together, around the largest part of the butt

Hips: _____

Measure right under the butt

Thigh Left: _____

Thigh Right: _____

SUGGESTED GROCERY LIST

Breakfast:

- ❑ Protein powder—whey, egg white, hemp, pea or rice protein
- ❑ Pasture-raised or free-range eggs
- ❑ Turkey bacon, uncured
- ❑ Natural and organic chicken and turkey sausage
- ❑ Greek yogurt (plain)
- ❑ Kefir, plain or flavored
- ❑ Steel cut oats or old fashioned oatmeal
- ❑ Low-fat cottage cheese
- ❑ Gluten-free baking mix for occasional pancakes or banana bread
- ❑ Frozen and fresh berries and fruit
- ❑ Cinnamon
- ❑ Almond butter
- ❑ Maple syrup
- ❑ Raw honey

Lunch and Dinner:

- ❑ Grass-fed meats, such as bison, lamb, and ground beef
- ❑ Ground turkey
- ❑ Free-range chicken breasts
- ❑ High omega-3 fish, such as wild salmon, sardines, and tuna
- ❑ Tempeh or tofu
- ❑ Garbanzo and black beans
- ❑ Spinach or other deep-colored greens
- ❑ Lettuce and mixed greens, such as romaine and arugula (not iceberg)
- ❑ Lemons, limes, oranges
- ❑ Grass-fed or raw milk cheese
- ❑ Goat's milk cheese
- ❑ Yams or sweet potatoes
- ❑ Broccoli, cauliflower, brussels sprouts, cabbage
- ❑ Yellow, green, and red peppers
- ❑ Quinoa
- ❑ Brown rice

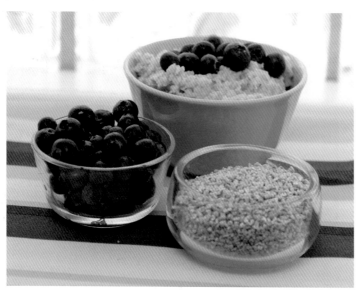

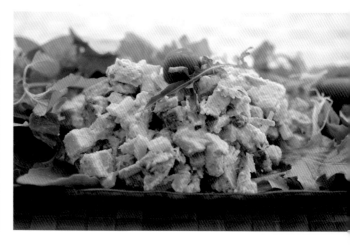

Snacks, Extras, and Desserts:

- ❏ Organic beef or turkey jerky
- ❏ Dry roasted almonds
- ❏ Pumpkin seeds
- ❏ Hummus and celery
- ❏ Brown rice crackers
- ❏ Olive and/or coconut oil
- ❏ Garlic and onions
- ❏ Ginger
- ❏ Parsley, dill, rosemary—fresh is best
- ❏ Ground or toasted flax seeds and chia seeds for shakes or oatmeal
- ❏ Pesto
- ❏ Miso
- ❏ Coconut ice cream
- ❏ Fresh berries

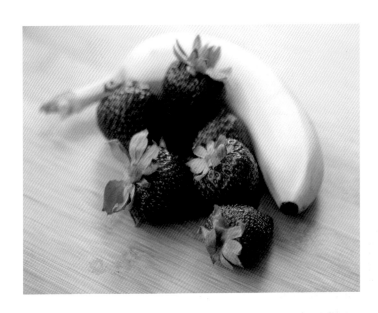

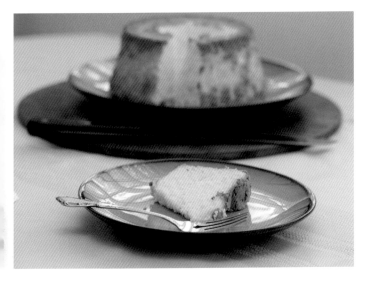

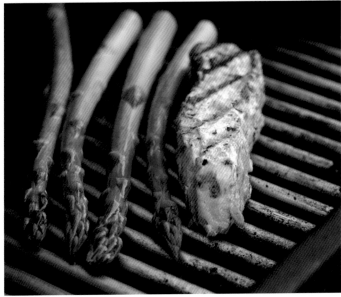

233

WEBSITES & ADDITIONAL READING

Tools for your Mind and Stress Reduction:

www.6weekbeachbody.com
www.thehotproject.com

Exercise Tools for Home, Gym, Office or Travel:

www.invisiblefitness.com

Calorie Counting Resources:

http://caloriecount.about.com
www.my-calorie-counter.com
www.myfooddiary.com
www.sparkpeople.com

Body Fat Calculator:

http://fitness.bizcalcs.com/Calculator.asp?Calc=Body-Fat-Navy

Find an acupuncturist:

www.acufinder.com
(and check with your health insurance for local providers in your area as well)

Author Recommended Websites:

Author's Book Site:
www.jjsabbook.com

Bodyblade:
http://bodyblade.com

Buy Local Produce:
http://www.localharvest.org

CoDynamics Pilates:
www.coe-dynamics.com

Dr. Jonny Bowden:
www.jonnybowden.com

Dr. Mercola:
www.mercola.com

Fitness Products:
www.fitnesswholesale.com

Fit2Love:
www.fit2love.info

Food Sensitivity Testing:
www.alcat.com

Gluten Free Info:
www.glutenfree.com
www.triumphdining.com

Gluten Sensitivity Testing:
www.enterolab.com

Healthy Body Club:
www.healthybodyclub.com.au

Hormone Testing:
www.labrix.com

Lucy:
www.lucy.com

Neurotransmitter Testing:
www.sanesco.net

Nourishing Wellness:
www.nourishingwellness.com

Restore Clothing:
www.restoreclothing.info

Slimware:
www.skinnyplates.com

Stroller Strides:
www.strollerstrides.com

9 Day Detox System:
www.jjsdetox.com

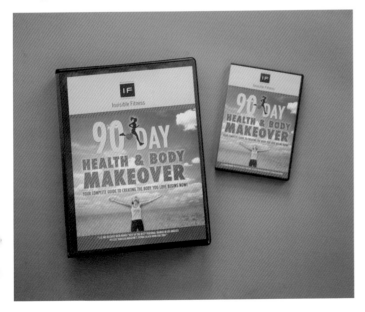

Recommended Books:

Ask and It Is Given: Learning to Manifest Your Desires by Esther and Jerry Hicks (The Teachings of Abraham). Hay House, 2005.

Breakthrough: Eight Steps to Wellness by Suzanne Somers. Three Rivers Press, 2009.

Fit 2 Love: How to Get Physically, Emotionally, and Spiritually Fit to Attract the Love of Your Life by JJ Flizanes. Bush Street Press, 2011.

Getting in the Gap by Dr. Wayne Dyer. Hay House, 2002.

Green for Life by Victoria Boutenko. Raw Family Publishing, 2005.

Knockout: Interviews with Doctors Who Are Curing Cancer—And How to Prevent Getting It in the First Place by Suzanne Somers. Crown Archetype, 2009.

The Paleo Diet: Lose Weight and Get Healthy by Eating the Food You Were Designed to Eat by Loren Cordain. Wiley, 2002.

The Power of Intention by Dr. Wayne Dyer. Hay House, 2005.

The 150 Healthiest Foods on Earth: The Surprising, Unbiased Truth About What You Should Eat and Why by Jonny Bowden Ph.D. C.N.S. Fair Winds Press, 2007.

You Can Heal Your Life by Louise L. Hay. Hay House, 1984.

5-Minute Diet Book by Ajay Rochester. New Holland Publishers, 2011.

GLOSSARY

GLOSSARY

Active Stretching: Using your own muscles to length other muscles without the help of an outside force. Using your hand to pull on your arm for a "better" stretch would be using an outside force to stretch which is not active but passive. Passive stretching can be dangerous and ineffective. A cat stretch is an active stretch because you contract your abs to stretch your back and you contract your back muscles to stretch your abs.

Aerobic Exercise: Also referred to as cardiovascular training (cardio). This type of exercise uses a low level of resistance with an extended duration such as fifteen minutes to several hours. Aerobic exercise conditions the heart and respiratory system.

Agonist: A muscle that causes specific movement via its own contraction. Agonists are also referred to as prime movers because they are primarily responsible for generating a specific movement.

Antagonist: A muscle that acts in opposition to the specific movement generated by the agonist.

Anterior: To the front; for example the anterior deltoid is on the front of your shoulder.

Biomechanics: Referring to the mechanics of the human body.

Bodyblade: A rapid-contraction training tool used to strengthen the core, increase balance, coordination and strength.

Body Composition: The measurement of what your bady is made of: fat, muscle, water, lean mass. Used to test mainly body fat and water.

Body-weight Exercises: Exercises that use a part or all of your body weight for resistance. Push-ups and sit-ups are examples of body-weight exercises.

Cable Crossover Machine: A training machine that uses cables to redirect gravity and create multiple exercises. These machines have many attachments and options for creating an exercise you may want.

Calorie: A calorie is the metric unit of heat measurement. Wh used in relation to nutrition, it refers to the energy value of food the amount of energy used when performing an exercise.

Carbohydrate: Foods that contain carbon, hydrogen and oxyg such as sugars, starches and cellulose. Fruits, vegetables, gra and starches are carbohydrates and get broken down to gluc in the body. Glucose is the body's main energy source like ga your car.

Cardiovascular Training: Also called aerobic exercise or cardio cular conditioning, see Aerobic Exercise.

Cortisol: An adrenal hormone produced by the adrenal cortex regulates carbohydrate metabolism and the immune system a maintains blood pressure. Often referred to as a stress hormone, v high or very low levels of cortisol can inhibit the body's ability recover and cause weight-loss resistance.

Cellulite: A fatty deposit causing a dimpled or uneven appe ance most commonly around the thighs and buttocks. Cellulit fat in between the layers of skin and can be found anywhere the body.

Cholesterol: A fat-based substance essential for cell health. Cho terol is produced in the body and absorbed from foods. Too mu cholesterol can build up on the artery walls, causing stroke and ot circulatory problems.

Concentric Contraction: A muscular contraction where the mus shortens as you move it.

Cross-training: A combination of two or more types of phys activity.

Delayed-onset Muscle Soreness: Discomfort or soreness felt the muscles worked twenty-four to seventy-two hours after exer ing. It is associated with muscle cell damage and micro-tears in muscle fibers.

Doorstop: An aid to using tubing to create exercises. Often included in the purchase of tubing, it is often a heavy material that is threaded in the door that has a piece of wood in it to secure it from coming through the door. Using a doorstop allows you to workout anywhere and safely secure the tubing in the door at any height to customize exercises for you.

Dumbbell: A weight that can be held in one hand.

Eccentric Contraction: A muscular contraction where the muscle lengthens as you move it and is usually the second action after a concentric contraction. The opposite muscle of the one doing a concentric contraction is also most likely experiencing an eccentric contraction.

Elliptical Trainer: A type of low-impact training machine used for cardiovascular exercise. It has a circular motion at the pedals and is often said to be a combination of a StairMaster and treadmill or a standing bicycle.

Endorphin: Naturally occurring neurotransmitters found in the brain and nervous system. Endorphins have opiate-like properties, relieving pain and creating a feeling of well-being.

Endurance Training: Exercising to increase stamina and endurance.

Extension: To straighten out, or move to a position of full length or to increase the angle between the bones.

External Rotation: Rotary motion away from the midline.

Fad Diet: Popular but scientifically unsound or unproven, fad diets promise quick results and are relatively easy to implement. They rarely promote sound weight loss and only work short-term, if at all.

Flexibility: The ability to move in a direction. Flexibility will be determined by the structure. Not all people are built the same and therefore will not "fold" the same. Factors that contribute to flexibility are muscle length, joint space, ligament length, bone length and the nervous systems connection to the muscle you want to move and the surrounding muscles.

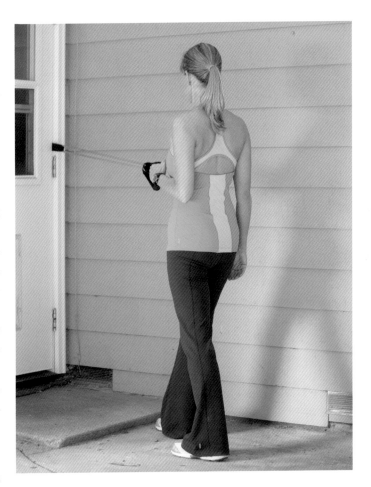

Flexion: The bending of a limb or joint to decrease the angle between the bones.

Food and Drug Administration (FDA): An agency of the Department of Health and Human Services of the U.S. government. It regulates the use of food, drugs, medical devices, and related products.

Free-motion Machines: An adjustable cable machine that uses two cables to create many different exercises for the whole body.

237

Free Weight: A weight, such as a barbell or dumbbell, that is not constrained or attached to another device.

Frontal Plane: Also called the coronal plane, this divides the body into front and back halves.

Heart Rate Monitor (HRM): An electrical device that measures your heart rate by sensing the electrical impulses produced by your heart. Heart rate monitors are usually incorporated in a wristwatch and use a chest strap to sense the impulses.

HDL: High-density lipoproteins (HDLs) enable your body to move fats and cholesterol within the bloodstream. They are also thought to remove damaging plaque from the artery walls, aiding in the prevention of heart disease.

Horizontal Plane: Also called the transverse plane, this divides the body horizontally into upper and lower halves.

Hormones: A naturally occurring chemical messenger that transports signals from one cell to another.

Hyperextension: The position of a joint or a part of the body extending beyond the normal range of motion.

Internal Rotation: Rotary motion toward the midline.

Isometric Exercise: A type of strength training in which you don't change the position of the exercising muscles during contraction. The exercise is done in a static position so that the muscles either work against an immovable object or are held in a static position against other muscles.

Lateral: Toward the outside or side of the body.

LDL: Low-density lipoproteins (LDLs) enable your body to move fats and cholesterol within the bloodstream. High levels of LDLs are an indicator of medical problems like heart disease.

Lean Body Mass: The amount of muscle in your body, especially skeletal muscle.

Massage: The practice of soft-tissue manipulation using press tension, motion, or vibration. Massage is used to work on musc tendons, ligaments, skin, joints, lymphatic vessels, and the gas intestinal system. It can be applied with the hands, fingers, elbo forearms, and feet.

Medial: Toward the midline or middle of the body.

Median Plane: Also called the sagittal plane, it divides the bo down the middle into left and right halves.

Metabolism, Metabolic Processes: Metabolism is the group chemical reactions that occur in your body to maintain life. Th metabolic processes allow you to grow and reproduce, maintain sues and organs, and function effectively.

Osteoporosis: Bone condition characterized by a decrease in d sity and an increase in porosity and brittleness.

Passive Stretching: Using an outside force to move your body i a position it cannot do by itself. Using a door frame, your body wei or someone else to stretch your muscle beyond the range of mot it could do alone can be dangerous and ineffective.

Pedometer: A small electronic device that can often measure spe distance, number of steps, and calories burned while walking or r ning depending on the model.

Planes of Motion: A system for describing the body's movem in three perpendicular planes—the frontal, lateral, and medial. planes of motion describe movement relative to your body at a n tral stance.

Plyometrics: A type of exercise training designed to produce f powerful movements and improve the functions of the nervous s tem. Plyometrics may include jumping, bounding, and hopping ex cises. Plyometrics can be dangerous on the joints if the body is prepared for the increase in intensity and speed.

Posterior: To the back; for example the posterior deltoid is on the back of your shoulder.

Prime Movers: The large muscles in your body that provide the bulk of the power when you perform a movement.

Prone: Lying down on your stomach with your face down.

Proprioception: The ability to sense the position, location, orientation, and movement of the body.

Protein: A complex organic compound essential for the chemical processes that sustain life. Dietary protein is found in foods such as meat, fish, and eggs.

Range of Motion: The distance between the fully flexed position and fully extended position of a joint or muscle group.

Reps: The number of repetitions of an exercise movement in a "set." One rep is a complete exercise cycle; for example one biceps curl.

Resistance Bands: Large elastic bands, often with handles, used as a total-body training system.

Resistance Exercise: See Resistance Training.

Resistance Training: A form of training in which muscular effort is performed against an opposing force. The goal of resistance training is to gradually and progressively overload the musculoskeletal system so it gets stronger.

Respiratory System: The body system for breathing. It includes the lungs and airways.

Set: A group of repeated exercises, or reps; for example, a set of twelve biceps curls.

Skeletal Muscle: The muscles that attach to bones, usually via tendons. Skeletal muscle is contracted voluntarily (by thinking about it), unlike cardiac (heart) muscle and the smooth muscle of the digestive tract that act without conscious thought.

Smith Machine: An apparatus that constrains a barbell to move only upward and downward. Some Smith machines allow limited forward and backward movement.

Spot Reducing: A mythical belief that it is possible to loose fat in an isolated area by exercising that particular area.

Stability Ball: An exercise ball, also known as a Swiss Ball, made of soft, durable plastic with a diameter of 35 to 85 centimeters (14 to 34 inches).

Stabilizer Muscles: The smaller peripheral muscles that provide stabilization and support for your joints and movements.

Strength Training: The use of resistance to build the strength, muscular endurance, and tone of skeletal muscles. There are many different methods of strength training

Superset: A training technique combining two or more consecutive exercises with little or no rest in between.

Supination: Rolling or rotating to the outside.

Supine: Lying on your back, face up.

Target Heart Rate Range: The minimum and maximum heart rate in beats per minute (BPM) between which you want to train. Target heart rate range varies depending on your training goals, your age and your fitness level.

Tubing: Elastic bands or tubes that can be used to build strength and muscle.

Unilateral: One side only.

Yoga: A system of exercises practiced as part of a Hindu philosophy to promote control of the body and mind. There are many variations and forms of yoga.

INDEX

INDEX

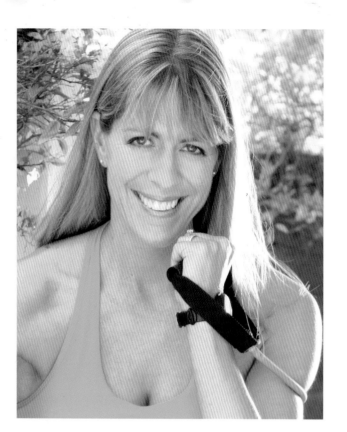

About the Author

JJ Flizanes, is the director of Invisible Fitness, a Beverly Hills, California–based business of health and well-being, and the creator of world-class fitness programs and routines. Author of *Fit 2 Love: How to Get Physically, Emotionally, and Spiritually Fit to Attract the Love of Your Life,* JJ was named by Elite Traveler Magazine as its 2007 Global Black Book pick of Best Personal Trainer in Los Angeles. In 2010 she was chosen by her peers as a finalist for IDEA Personal Trainer of the Year. JJ is certified by the National Academy of Sports Medicine and has also served as Continuing Education Provider. She has lectured for The Learning Annex and as a featured speaker for New York Times bestselling author T. Harv Ecker's Peak Potentials seminars as well as some corporate clients including Pacific Gas and Electric, Hanson Engineering, and Jostens Inc. She has been featured in many magazines, including, *Woman's Health, Muscle and Fitness HERS, Elegant Bride, Fitness Magazine,* and *E Pregnancy* Magazine. Her television appearances include LA's KTLA, CBS, and NBC. Visit her at invisiblefitness.com.

About the Photographer

Starla Fortunato continues to photograph some of the biggest names in the entertainment industry. Her uncompromising dedication to finding beauty in every face is becoming legendary. This is because Starla believes that "every face has a sublime angle", and she's committed to unlocking each client's most attractive features to produce powerful portraiture. Her unfettered images, both soulful and gorgeous, have appeared in *Venice Magazine, Glamour, TV Guide, Angeleno, Los Angeles Times, Teen Vogue* and other publications. Fortunato contributed an impressive mix of stunning celebrity portraits for Morgan Freeman's book project "Morgan Freeman and Friends". Starla enjoys collaborative work with creative people. Her studio is located in Hollywood California and she travels globally for assignments.

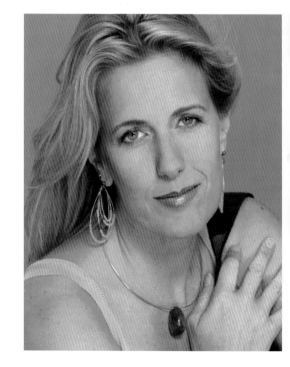